HOLISTIC LIVING *for* FITNESS

A Mindful Approach to Workouts, Meal Planning, and Lasting Weight Loss in a Hectic World

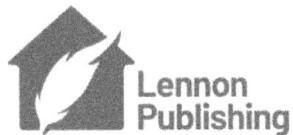

Copyright © 2025 by Lennon Publishing

All rights reserved.

No portion of this book may be reproduced in any form without written permission from the publisher or author, except as permitted by U.S. copyright law.

This publication is designed to provide accurate and authoritative information in regard to the subject matter covered. It is sold with the understanding that neither the author nor the publisher is engaged in rendering legal, investment, accounting or other professional services. While the publisher and author have used their best efforts in preparing this book, they make no representations or warranties with respect to the accuracy or completeness of the contents of this book and specifically disclaim any implied warranties of merchantability or fitness for a particular purpose. No warranty may be created or extended by sales representatives or written sales materials. The advice and strategies contained herein may not be suitable for your situation. You should consult with a professional when appropriate. Neither the publisher nor the author shall be liable for any loss of profit or any other commercial damages, including but not limited to special, incidental, consequential, personal, or other damages.

Second edition 2025

Contents

Note To The Reader   1

Introduction   2

1. Embracing the Mind-Body Connection   5
    Understanding Holistic Fitness
    The Science of Mindfulness in Exercise
    Cultivating Awareness in Movement
    Breathing Techniques for Mental Clarity
    Body Scanning for Stress Reduction
    Integrating Mindfulness into Daily Routines

2. Mindful Nutrition Essentials   29
    Building a Balanced Plate with Intention
    Recognizing Hunger and Fullness Cues
    Savoring Food: Techniques for Slowing Down
    Emotional Eating: Identifying and Overcoming Triggers
    Sustainable Meal Planning and Prep

3. Personalized Fitness for Every Lifestyle   51
    Time-Efficient Workouts for Busy Schedules
    Functional Fitness for Everyday Life
    Low-Impact Exercises for All Ages
    Incorporating Yoga and Stretching for Flexibility

Strength Training for Beginners

4. Creating Lasting Habits　　　　　　　　　　　　73
    Habit Stacking for Seamless Integration
    Overcoming Barriers to Change
    Setting Realistic and Achievable Goals
    Maintaining Motivation Through Accountability
    Tracking Progress and Celebrating Milestones

5. Mindful Living and Stress Management　　　　　91
    Mindfulness Techniques for Stress Relief
    The Power of Meditation in Daily Life
    Prioritizing Sleep for Optimal Health
    Digital Detox: Reclaiming Your Mind for Mindfulness
    The Impact of Digital Overload
    The Benefits of a Digital Detox
    Practical Steps for a Digital Detox
    Reclaiming Balance and Presence
    Cultivating a Positive Mindset

6. Ethical and Environmental Considerations　　107
    Interactive Journal: Ethical Shopping Checklist
    Navigating Plant-Based Nutrition
    Balancing Ethical Eating with Personal Health
    Reducing Food Waste: Practical Tips
    Sustainable Sourcing: Making Informed Choices
    The Environmental Impact of Dietary Choices

7. Interactive Journaling for Self-Discovery　　125
    Journaling Prompts for Mindful Eating
    Tracking Emotional Well-Being

    Visualizing Your Health Goals
    Gratitude Practices for Positivity
    Creating a Personalized Wellness Journal

8. Enhancing Your Wellness Journey with Technology   144
    Interactive Journal: Fitness App Evaluation Checklist
    Digital Tools for Tracking Nutrition
    Online Communities for Support and Motivation
    Virtual Workouts: Finding What Works for You
    Mindfulness Apps to Enhance Meditation
    Balancing Screen Time with Mindful Living

9. Conclusion   163

Extended Edition: Travel-Friendly Workouts   166
    Sample Travel Day Plan

Bonus Chapter: Fitness Myths Debunked   173
Separating Fact from Fiction

References   182

Note To The Reader

Thank you for picking up the Second Edition of *Holistic Living for Fitness: A Mindful Approach to Workouts, Meal Planning, and Lasting Weight Loss in a Hectic World.*

We loved how you embraced the **Bonus Chapter: Fitness Myths Debunked** in the first edition, so we've gone a step further with an **Extended-Edition Bonus Chapter: Travel-Friendly Workouts**. Inside, you'll find five zero-equipment circuits to keep you moving anywhere—from hotel rooms to park benches.

If you're returning for a refresher, welcome back—you helped inspire these new routines. If this is your first time through, get ready for playful challenges, fresh insights and easy-to-follow rituals that fit right into your busy life.

Let's hit the road (and the mat)!

Second Edition, 2025

Introduction

You're running late for work, juggling a phone call and a half-eaten sandwich, and the idea of fitting in a workout today seems laughable. Sound familiar? For many of us, life feels like a never-ending race against the clock. We're trying to balance our careers, families, and social lives, often at the expense of our health and well-being. I've been there too, caught in the hustle, feeling like there's never enough time for self-care.

This book is here to change that narrative. The primary goal is to empower you to achieve holistic wellness through mindful nutrition, exercise, and sustainable lifestyle changes. Think of it as your friendly guide, offering practical advice and helping you build habits that last. No more fads or quick fixes—just real solutions that fit into your busy life.

What makes this book unique is its interactive approach. It's not just a read-and-forget kind of book. It's a guided journal designed for active participation. You'll find prompts for self-reflection, goal setting, and even curated music suggestions to make your journey more enjoyable. By the end of each chapter, you'll have a personalized map of your own wellness path.

Who will benefit from this journey? Whether you're navigating the demands of a burgeoning career, managing the whirlwind of parenthood, or adjusting to a new chapter in your life, this guide is crafted with you in mind. You prioritize personal development and seek authentic, feasible strategies for self-care amidst a schedule brimming with obligations.

The themes we'll explore together are interconnected: mindful eating, holistic fitness, and sustainable weight loss. Each plays a crucial role in your journey toward comprehensive well-being. Mindful eating encourages you to appreciate your food and understand its impact on your body. Holistic fitness focuses on exercises that you enjoy and can maintain. Sustainable weight loss is about making changes that stick, without feeling deprived.

I know the struggle of sifting through conflicting health advice. It can be confusing and overwhelming, especially when time and motivation are in short supply. This book addresses these common pain points by offering clear, actionable solutions. It's about cutting through the noise and finding what truly works for you.

Let's talk about how this book is structured. We'll start with foundational concepts that set the stage for your wellness journey. Each chapter progresses to practical applications, complete with journal prompts and exercises to encourage self-discovery and habit formation. You'll learn how to integrate these practices into your daily routine effortlessly.

This guide is designed to be practical and accessible. The advice here is easy to follow and meant to be adapted to your lifestyle, regardless of your current fitness level or experience with wellness practices. Whether you're just starting or looking to deepen your current routine, you'll find something valuable here.

As you engage with this book, you'll begin to see a transformation. You'll discover that holistic health is not only attainable but also empowering. Mindful living will become second nature, and you'll feel more balanced and energized. You'll gain the confidence to take control of your health in a way that feels right for you.

So, let's embark on this journey together. You have the tools you need within these pages to create a life that supports your well-being. Take a deep breath, turn the page, and step into a world where health and happiness coexist, even amidst the busyness of life.

Chapter 1

Embracing the Mind-Body Connection

You know those days when your body feels like it's on autopilot, ticking off tasks without a second thought? You might be checking emails during breakfast, squeezing in a quick workout between meetings, and mindlessly snacking while trying to meet deadlines. We've all had days like that, feeling like we're just going through the motions without being truly present. This chapter invites you to press pause on that chaos. It's a gentle nudge to reconnect with yourself—not just physically, but mentally and emotionally too. It's about finding harmony in a world that often feels anything but balanced. Here, we'll explore how embracing the connection between your mind and body can transform your approach to fitness and wellness.

Understanding Holistic Fitness

Holistic fitness is not just another trend. It's a comprehensive approach that emphasizes the interconnectedness of your body, mind, and inner self. Imagine a fitness regime where strength, mental clarity, and emotional resilience are equally prioritized. This approach is about achieving harmony across all aspects of health, rather than focusing solely on physical appearance or performance. It's about recognizing that your mental and emotional well-being are just as important as your physical strength. By integrating body, mind, and spirit, you create a balanced lifestyle that nurtures every part of you. This balance can lead to lasting health benefits, helping you navigate life with a sense of calm and purpose.

Traditional fitness models often fall short when it comes to addressing overall well-being. They tend to overemphasize physical appearance, promoting the idea that fitness is solely about achieving a certain look. This focus can neglect the mental health components that are crucial for sustained wellness. When exercise becomes solely about aesthetics, it can lead to burnout, dissatisfaction, and a disconnect between body and mind. Holistic fitness, on the other hand, promotes a balanced approach that considers the whole person. It encourages you to move with intention, focusing on how exercise makes you feel rather than just how it makes you look.

Balance is the cornerstone of holistic fitness. It involves giving equal importance to strength, flexibility, and endurance. Each component contributes to overall health and wellness, ensuring that your body is well-rounded and capable of handling various physical demands. Strength training builds muscle and bone density, while flexibility exercises like yoga improve range of motion and prevent injuries. Endurance activities, such as running or cycling, enhance cardiovascular health and stamina. Together, these elements create a fitness routine that supports your body's needs, helping you feel strong, agile, and resilient.

Mindfulness plays a crucial role in achieving a holistic fitness regime. Mindful movement practices encourage you to be present during exercise, focusing on the sensations in your body and the rhythm of your breath. This awareness helps you connect with your body on a deeper level, enhancing the effectiveness of your workouts. Mindfulness also promotes mental clarity, which is essential for staying motivated and committed to your fitness goals. When you exercise with mindfulness, you cultivate a sense of inner peace and focus that extends beyond the gym. It becomes a practice that nourishes your mind and spirit, leaving you feeling rejuvenated and centered.

Reflection Journal

Consider your current fitness routine. Reflect on how much of it focuses solely on physical appearance versus overall well-being. Jot down any changes you'd like to make to incorporate more mindfulness and balance. How can you better integrate strength, flexibility, and endurance into your routine? What small steps can you take to ensure your workouts nourish both your body and mind? This exercise is a starting point for embracing holistic fitness, helping you create a plan that aligns with your values and lifestyle.

Reflection on My Current Fitness Routine Take a moment to reflect: How much of your current routine is focused on physical appearance? How much supports your overall well-being? Are you satisfied with the balance?

My thoughts:

Changes I'd Like to Make Think about how you can bring more mindfulness and balance into your routine. What areas feel neglected? How can you shift your focus to activities that nourish both body and mind?

I'd like to:

Building Strength, Flexibility, and Endurance Consider ways to incorporate these three pillars into your fitness plan. What activities feel enjoyable and sustainable for you?

- **Strength:**

- **Flexibility:**

- **Endurance:**

Small Steps Toward Holistic Fitness What small, actionable changes can you start today or this week? Reflect on ways to make your workouts more intentional and aligned with your values.

My next steps:

Final Thoughts How do you feel after reflecting on your fitness routine? What motivates you to make these changes? What impact do you hope this holistic approach will have on your life?

Closing thoughts:

Music Suggestion Enhance your reflection or workout experience with music that inspires mindfulness and energy. Try:

- **Instrumental Focus:** *Weightless* by Marconi Union

- **Mindful Energy:** *Aloha Ke Akua* by Nahko and Medicine for the People

- **Strength & Power:** *Eye of the Tiger* by Survivor

- **Relaxation & Stretching:** *Clair de Lune* by Debussy

The Science of Mindfulness in Exercise

Imagine you're in the middle of a workout, your mind racing with thoughts of unfinished tasks and looming deadlines. Yet, as you settle into the rhythm of your movements, something shifts. You focus on your breath, the sensation of your muscles contracting and releasing, and the gentle beat of your heart. This is mindfulness in exercise, a practice that transforms a routine workout into a meditative experience. Scientifically, mindfulness during exercise reduces cortisol levels, the notorious stress hormone that often keeps us in a state of constant tension. Lowering cortisol not only eases stress but also enhances focus and concentration, allowing you to be fully present in each movement. When your mind is clear, your workouts become more efficient, and you find yourself moving with purpose rather than obligation. This enhanced focus creates a positive loop, improving your muscle relaxation and overall performance. With each mindful breath, you become more in tune with your body's needs, fostering a sense of calm and control.

On the neurological front, mindfulness in exercise plays a fascinating role. Engaging in mindful practices can increase neuroplasticity, the brain's ability to adapt and reorganize itself. This adaptability translates into enhanced memory and learning, crucial benefits for those of us juggling countless responsibilities. Picture your brain as a muscle—it strengthens with use, becoming more adept at handling complex tasks and retaining new information. When you integrate mindfulness into your exercise routine, you're not just training your body but also sharpening your brain. Studies have shown that mindfulness-based interventions can significantly improve cognitive performance, helping you tackle daily challenges with newfound clarity and creativity. As your brain becomes more efficient, you might notice an improvement in decision-making and problem-solving, skills that are invaluable in both personal and professional settings.

Mental health, too, reaps the rewards of mindfulness in exercise. Regular practice can lead to a reduction in symptoms of anxiety and depression, offering a natural and empowering way to manage mental health. By focusing on the present moment, you create a mental space free from worry and fear. This presence allows you to connect with your emotions, understand them, and let go of those that do not serve you. Engaging in mindful workouts can become a form of moving meditation, where the act of exercising becomes a powerful tool for nurturing mental well-being.

As mindfulness practices take root, you'll likely experience an increase in self-compassion and acceptance, fostering a healthier relationship with yourself and your body.

So, how do we bring mindfulness into our exercise routines? Mindful yoga sequences are a brilliant place to start. Yoga emphasizes breath control and awareness of the body, encouraging you to move with intention. Each pose becomes an opportunity to explore your body's capabilities and limitations without judgment. Focused breathing, a core component of yoga, further enhances the connection between mind and body. Alternatively, consider incorporating breathing-focused aerobic activities, such as walking or running, where the rhythm of your breath guides each step. These activities encourage a meditative state, allowing you to immerse yourself in the flow of movement and breath. The goal is not to achieve perfection but to cultivate a practice that supports both physical fitness and mental clarity.

Mindful Movement Journal

Next time you head out for a run or walk, try this mindful exercise: as you begin, focus on the sensation of your feet touching the ground. Feel the texture beneath you and the rhythm of your steps. Gradually bring your attention to your breath, matching its pace with the movement. If your mind starts to wander, gently bring it back to the present moment. Notice the sights, sounds, and sensations around you. This simple exercise transforms a routine activity into an opportunity for mindfulness, helping you connect with yourself and the world in a meaningful way.

Reflection on My Current Movement Practice Take a moment to consider your usual approach to walking or running. How present are you during these activities? Do you often find your mind wandering, or are you fully engaged with the experience?

My thoughts:

Intentions for Mindful Movement Think about how you can bring more mindfulness to your next walk or run. What sensations, rhythms, or surroundings would you like to focus on?

I'd like to focus on:

Mindful Movement Exercise The next time you go for a walk or run, try the following steps:

- **Feet:** Focus on the sensation of your feet touching the ground. What does the texture beneath you feel like? *My experience:*

- **Breath:** Bring attention to your breath. Can you match its pace with your steps? *My experience:*

- **Mindfulness:** If your thoughts wander, gently guide

them back to the present. Notice the sights, sounds, and sensations around you. *My experience:*

Small Steps to Make This a Habit What can you do to integrate this practice into your routine? How can you remind yourself to stay mindful during movement?

My next steps:

Final Thoughts How did this exercise make you feel? What insights or feelings came up during your mindful movement?

Closing thoughts:

Music Suggestion Enhance your mindful movement with music that complements your pace and helps you stay present:

- **For a Calm Walk:** *River Flows in You* by Yiruma

- **For an Energizing Run:** *Adventure of a Lifetime* by Coldplay

- **For Nature Walks:** *Morning Mood* by Edvard Grieg

- **For Focus and Grounding:** *Bloom* by ODESZA

Cultivating Awareness in Movement

When was the last time you truly paid attention to how your body moved? Maybe you were rushing through a workout, barely noticing how your muscles engaged and released. Awareness in movement invites you to change that perspective. It's about consciously engaging your muscles and paying attention to your form and posture. This level of awareness can transform exercise from a monotonous task to a mindful practice. By noticing the way your body moves, you create a deeper connection with it, enhancing the effectiveness of your workouts. It's like shifting from autopilot to manual mode, where each movement becomes intentional and meaningful.

Developing this awareness requires practice, but the benefits are well worth the effort. One technique is body scanning during workouts. This involves mentally checking in with different parts of your body as you move, noticing any tension or discomfort. It's about being present in each moment, focusing on the sensation of your muscles contracting and relaxing. Visualization exercises can also enhance awareness. Picture the muscles you're working, visualize their movement and imagine the energy flowing through them. These techniques help you engage more deeply with your body, improving your form and alignment.

Increased movement awareness can prevent injuries and enhance performance. Proper alignment and posture reduce the risk of strains and sprains, allowing you to exercise safely and effectively. When you're aware of how your body moves, you can make adjustments that prevent overexertion and imbalances. This awareness also enhances proprioception, your body's ability to sense its position and movement in space. Improved proprioception means greater balance and coordination, helping you move with confidence and precision.

Consider incorporating exercises that focus on building awareness into your routine. Tai Chi, for example, is a practice that emphasizes slow, deliberate movements, promoting balance and control. Each movement flows into the next, encouraging you to focus on the present moment and the sensations in your body. Pilates is another excellent choice, as it emphasizes core awareness and alignment. The controlled movements require you to engage your muscles intentionally, fostering a deep connection between your mind and body.

Visualization Journal

Try this visualization exercise during your next workout. As you perform each movement, close your eyes for a moment and imagine the muscles you're engaging. Visualize them contracting and releasing, picture the energy flowing through them, and focus on the sensations in your body. This technique helps you tune into your body's needs, enhancing your awareness and improving your performance.

Reflection on My Mind-Body Connection Think about how connected you feel to your body during workouts. Do you often focus on the movements and sensations, or are you distracted by other thoughts?

My thoughts:

Intentions for Visualization Consider how incorporating visualization can improve your awareness and performance. What aspects of your workout do you want to focus on more deeply?

I'd like to focus on:

Visualization Exercise During your next workout, follow these steps to engage in visualization:

- **Close Your Eyes Momentarily:** As you perform each movement, take a moment to close your eyes (if it's safe to do so).*What I noticed:*

- **Visualize the Muscles Engaging:** Imagine the specific muscles you're using, contracting and releasing with each motion. *What I felt:*

- **Picture Energy Flowing:** Envision energy coursing through your body, fueling your movements and enhancing your strength. *My experience:*

- **Focus on Sensations:** Pay attention to the feelings in your body—the stretch, tension, and release. *My sensations:*

Small Steps to Make This a Habit How can you regularly incorporate visualization into your workouts? What reminders or tools could help you stay mindful?

My next steps:

Final Thoughts Reflect on how this visualization exercise impacted your workout. Did it change the way you experienced your movements? How did it affect your focus or performance?

Closing thoughts:

Music Suggestion Pair your visualization exercise with music that enhances focus and body awareness:

- **For Deep Focus:** *Weightless* by Marconi Union

- **For Slow, Controlled Movements:** *Nuvole Bianche* by

Ludovico Einaudi

- **For Energized Visualization:** *On Top of the World* by Imagine Dragons

- **For Centered Strength:** *Rise* by Hans Zimmer

Cultivating awareness in movement is about more than just exercise. It's a practice that extends into everyday life, helping you move through the world with intention and grace. Whether you're walking to work, lifting groceries, or playing with your kids, this awareness invites you to be present in each moment. It encourages you to appreciate the capabilities of your body and the joy of movement, creating a sense of gratitude and connection.

Breathing Techniques for Mental Clarity

Ever notice how a few deep breaths can change your entire perspective on a stressful situation? There's more to it than just a temporary sense of calm. The way we breathe affects our mental clarity and focus. When you take a deep breath, you're not just filling your lungs with air. You're oxygenating your brain, which is crucial for clear thinking and decision-making. This simple act also calms the nervous system by activating the parasympathetic nervous system, which is responsible for resting and digesting. It's like hitting the reset button for your mind, helping to clear away the fog that stress and anxiety often bring.

Let's explore some specific breathing exercises that can help enhance this mental clarity. Diaphragmatic breathing, or deep belly breathing, is a powerful technique. To try it, place one hand on your chest and the other on your belly. As you inhale deeply through your nose, your belly should rise more than your chest. This technique encourages full oxygen exchange, slows the heartbeat, and can lower or stabilize blood pressure. Another effective method is the 4-7-8 breathing technique. Start by breathing in quietly through your nose for four seconds, hold the breath for seven seconds, and then exhale completely through your mouth for eight seconds. This exercise is known to calm the mind, reduce anxiety, and help you fall asleep faster.

Breathing correctly can significantly reduce stress. When you're stressed, your body tends to take shallow, rapid breaths. This kind of breathing signals the fight-or-flight response, keeping the body in a state of alertness. By practicing proper breathing techniques, you can reverse this response, reducing physical tension and lowering your heart rate. It's amazing how something as simple as altering your breath can bring about such profound changes. Try these techniques next time you feel overwhelmed, and notice the difference in how your body responds to stress.

Breath control is not just about mental clarity; it also plays a crucial role in physical performance. Athletes and fitness enthusiasts know the importance of breathing techniques for improving endurance and efficiency. When you manage your breath, you optimize oxygen delivery to your muscles, which increases endurance and performance. Think of it like ensuring a steady flow of fuel to an engine. Efficient oxygen use means you can sustain activity for longer periods without exhaustion. Whether you're running a marathon or simply going for a brisk walk, mastering these techniques can give you that extra boost.

Breathing Journal

Try incorporating a simple breathing exercise into your daily routine. Set aside a few minutes each morning to practice diaphragmatic breathing. As you wake up, sit comfortably and close your eyes. Focus on taking deep, slow breaths, letting your mind clear as you inhale and exhale. This small practice can set a positive tone for the rest of your day, enhancing your focus and reducing stress. Remember, your breath is a powerful tool for achieving mental clarity and balance, so make it a part of your wellness toolkit.

Reflection on My Current Breathing Habits How often do you pay attention to your breath throughout the day? Do you notice any connection between your breathing and your stress or focus levels?

Intentions for Mindful Breathing What benefits do you hope to gain from practicing diaphragmatic breathing? How can this exercise support your overall well-being?

Breathing Exercise Incorporate this practice into your routine:

- **Start the Day with Breath:** Sit comfortably and close your eyes.

- **Focus on Your Breathing:** Take deep, slow breaths, feeling your diaphragm expand as you inhale and contract as you exhale.

- **Clear Your Mind:** Let go of any thoughts and simply be present with each breath.

Small Steps to Build a Habit How can you make this breathing exercise a consistent part of your day? What reminders or adjustments to your schedule might help?

Final Thoughts How did you feel after practicing this exercise? Did it impact your focus, mood, or stress levels? How might regular practice enhance your day-to-day life?

Music Suggestion Pair your breathing exercise with calming music to deepen the relaxation:

- **For Calm and Centering:** *Quiet Resource* by Liquid Mind

- **For Gentle Mornings:** *Prelude in E Minor* by Chopin

- **For Stress Reduction:** *Breathe* by Moby

Body Scanning for Stress Reduction

Picture yourself lying comfortably on your back, eyes gently closed, as you begin to tune into the rhythm of your breath. This simple yet profound practice is known as body scanning, a mindfulness meditation technique that encourages you to scan your body for any signs of pain, tension, or anything that feels out of the ordinary. Body scanning invites you to explore the connection between physical sensations and your mental state, fostering a sense of awareness that often gets lost in the hustle of daily life. By gradually shifting your attention from one part of your body to another, you cultivate a deeper understanding of how stress manifests physically. This awareness is the first step towards releasing chronic tension and promoting relaxation.

To begin, find a quiet space where you won't be disturbed. Lie down on a comfortable surface, such as a yoga mat or your bed, and close your eyes. Start by taking a few deep breaths, allowing your body to settle into relaxation. Slowly direct your attention to your toes, noticing any sensations without judgment. Perhaps you feel warmth, tingling, or tension. With each exhale, imagine any tension melting away. Gradually move your focus upward, from your feet to your ankles, calves, knees, and so on, until you reach the top of your head. As you scan each area, acknowledge any sensations you encounter, sending a breath of relaxation to those areas. The goal isn't to change anything but to simply notice and accept what is present.

Regular practice of body scanning can lead to significant stress reduction over time. By consistently checking in with your body, you train yourself to recognize and release tension before it becomes chronic. This practice enhances your relaxation response, a state where your body can restore itself and heal. The more you engage in body scanning, the more adept you become at recognizing early signs of stress, allowing you to take proactive steps to manage it. Imagine being able to catch yourself before stress spirals out of control, simply by tuning into the language of your body. This kind of self-awareness is empowering, giving you the tools to navigate stress with grace and confidence.

Body scanning is versatile and can be incorporated into various contexts throughout your day. Consider using it during the cool-down phase of your workout, when your body is already in a relaxed state and receptive to mindfulness. As you transition from movement to stillness, take a few minutes to scan your body, acknowledging the work it has done and releasing any residual tension. Alternatively, make body scanning a part of your daily mindfulness practice. Set aside a few moments each morning or evening to reconnect with your body, allowing this practice to become a soothing ritual that anchors your day. Whether you're winding down after a long day or preparing for the challenges ahead, body scanning offers a moment of peace and introspection.

Incorporating body scanning into your routine doesn't require any special equipment or expertise. It's a practice that meets you where you are, inviting you to pause and listen to the wisdom of your body. As you cultivate this awareness, you'll find that the boundaries between your physical sensations and mental states blur, revealing the intricate connection between body and mind. This practice not only reduces stress but also deepens your relationship with yourself, fostering a sense of compassion and understanding. As you continue to explore body scanning, you'll discover its potential to transform your experience of stress, guiding you towards a more mindful and balanced life.

Integrating Mindfulness into Daily Routines

Imagine waking up and feeling like you're fully present with each moment. The hum of the morning bustle doesn't overwhelm you but instead feels like a gentle reminder that you're alive. Mindfulness can bring this sense of presence and awareness into our daily routines. It's about creating habits that support mental and emotional well-being, allowing us to navigate life's challenges with grace. Integrating mindfulness into everyday life isn't about making drastic changes. It's about embedding small, consistent practices that sustain us, providing continuous support for our mental and emotional health. When mindfulness becomes a part of our daily routine, it lays the foundation for sustainable habits that foster holistic wellness.

Incorporating mindfulness doesn't have to be complicated. It can begin with mindful eating practices during meals. This means truly tasting and savoring each bite, paying attention to flavors and textures without distraction. By slowing down and engaging with your food, you create a moment of connection with yourself, turning an everyday activity into a mindful experience. Another simple yet profound practice is gratitude. Taking a moment each day to acknowledge what you're grateful for can shift your perspective and foster a positive mindset. It could be something as small as the warmth of your morning coffee or the smile of a loved one. These acts of mindfulness anchor us in the present, reminding us of the abundance in our lives.

The benefits of consistent mindfulness are profound. Regular practice can improve emotional regulation, helping us respond to situations with calm and clarity rather than reacting impulsively. It enhances overall satisfaction and well-being, allowing us to appreciate life's small joys and navigate challenges with resilience. As mindfulness becomes a regular practice, it cultivates a sense of peace and contentment that permeates every aspect of our lives. We begin to notice the beauty in the ordinary and find happiness in simplicity, creating a ripple effect that positively influences our relationships and interactions.

To enhance your mindfulness journey, explore the array of mindfulness tools and resources available. Apps designed for beginners feature guided meditations and timely reminders, serving as an invaluable aid to maintain consistency in your practice. These digital companions provide a solid foundation, guiding you gently into the realm of mindfulness. Additionally, recordings of guided meditations present another avenue to deepen your practice, offering expert-led instructions that you can follow at your own pace. Regardless of how much time you can dedicate—be it a brief five-minute pause or an extended hour-long session—these resources seamlessly integrate into your daily routine, ensuring mindfulness is both accessible and practical for your lifestyle.

As you integrate mindfulness into your routine, you'll find that it becomes a natural part of your day, like brushing your teeth or having your morning coffee. It's about creating a rhythm that aligns with your lifestyle, making mindfulness a seamless part of who you are. Over time, mindfulness transforms from a practice into a way of being, enriching your life with presence and purpose. You'll notice a shift in how you perceive and interact with the world, feeling more grounded and connected.

Incorporating mindfulness into daily life doesn't require perfection. It's a journey of exploration, where each day offers an opportunity to learn and grow. Some days you may feel deeply connected, while others may be more challenging. Embrace each experience with curiosity and compassion, knowing that mindfulness is a practice that evolves with you. As you continue to cultivate mindfulness, you'll find that it enhances your overall well-being, providing a steady anchor amidst the ebb and flow of life. Embrace mindfulness as a companion on your path, guiding you towards a life of balance and fulfillment.

Chapter 2

Mindful Nutrition Essentials

Sitting at your desk, the laptop's glow reflects in the room, accompanied by the relentless ticking of the clock. Hours have slipped away, and you find yourself reaching for another snack on autopilot. This scenario is all too familiar for many of us—eating without awareness, hardly noticing as the food quickly vanishes. This habit of mindless eating, driven by convenience rather than genuine enjoyment, is a pattern many fall into. However, it's possible to rewrite this script. Mindful eating presents a compelling alternative, centering on the full sensory experience of our meals rather than solely their calorie content or nutritional value. This method encourages a full engagement with what we eat, taking the time to relish each bite and truly appreciate the taste and texture of our food. It transforms eating from a routine task into an act of mindfulness, creating a moment to connect deeply with our food and ourselves, and nurturing a more positive relationship with both.

Mindful eating is a practice that emphasizes awareness, encouraging you to slow down and truly notice what you're eating. Unlike traditional eating patterns, which often prioritize speed and efficiency, mindful eating asks you to pause and engage your senses. It's about tuning into the taste, smell, and even sound of your food. This practice helps reduce mindless eating habits, which can be unhealthy and often lead to overeating. When meals become an automatic, hurried act, you lose the ability to recognize when you're truly satisfied, leading to unnecessary consumption. Mindful eating, on the other hand, cultivates a sense of presence, allowing you to enjoy your food without distraction and recognize when you've had enough.

The benefits of mindful eating extend beyond mere enjoyment. One significant advantage is improved digestion. When you eat slowly, your body has more time to signal fullness, and your digestive system can process food more effectively. This slower pace can reduce discomfort and bloating, common issues when meals are rushed. Mindful eating also leads to greater satisfaction with smaller portions. By paying attention to the experience of eating, you become more attuned to your body's signals, realizing you need less to feel content. This can naturally lead to healthier portion control and a more balanced diet.

So how do you start practicing mindful eating? It begins with setting a calm, distraction-free environment. Create a space where you can focus solely on your meal, free from the usual interruptions of screens and noise. Before you take your first bite, ask yourself a few questions: Why are you eating right now? Are you truly hungry, or are you eating out of habit or emotion? Consider the nutritional value of what you're about to consume. These questions help ground you in the present moment and align your eating with your body's actual needs.

Mindful eating can be seamlessly integrated into various aspects of your daily life. Take snacking during work breaks, for example. Instead of mindlessly munching while checking emails, dedicate a few minutes to really taste your snack. Notice the texture, the flavors, and how it makes you feel. This practice transforms a quick snack into a nourishing pause, recharging your body and mind. Dining out is another opportunity to practice mindfulness. When you're at a restaurant, take a moment before eating to admire the presentation of your dish. Engage with each bite, savoring the chef's craft, and enjoy the company of those around you without rushing through the meal.

Reflection Journal

Consider your last meal. Reflect on how you approached it—were you mindful or distracted? What was the environment like? Take a moment to jot down your thoughts and any changes you'd like to implement. How can you make your next meal a more mindful experience? What steps will you take to ensure you're present, engaged, and truly enjoying your food? This reflection is the first step in cultivating a mindful eating practice that supports both your physical health and emotional well-being.

Reflection on My Last Meal Think about your most recent meal. Were you mindful or distracted? What was the environment like? How did you feel during and after the meal?

Changes I'd Like to Make Consider how you can approach your next meal more mindfully. What adjustments to your environment, mindset, or habits would help you stay present and engaged?

Creating a Mindful Eating Practice As you plan your next meal, think about the following:

- **Preparation:** How can you create a calm and inviting space for your meal?

- **Engagement:** What can you focus on while eating (e.g., flavors, textures, gratitude)?

- **Presence:** What distractions can you minimize to stay fully in the moment?

Small Steps to Build the Habit What small, actionable steps can you take to incorporate mindful eating into your daily routine?

Final Thoughts How does reflecting on your eating habits make you feel? What benefits do you hope to gain by cultivating a mindful eating practice?

Music Suggestion Enhance your mindful eating experience with soothing background music:

- **For Calm and Relaxation:** *Canon in D* by Pachelbel

- **For a Peaceful Atmosphere:** *Pure Shores* by All Saints

- **For Gratitude and Reflection:** *Thank You* by Alanis Morissette

Building a Balanced Plate with Intention

Creating a balanced plate isn't just about filling your plate with random foods or sticking strictly to calorie counts. It's about ensuring that each meal is a harmonious blend of nutrients that cater to your body's needs. Imagine your plate as a canvas, and you're the artist. On one side, you have proteins—lean meats, fish, beans, or tofu—that work to build and repair tissues. A quarter of your plate should hold these powerhouses. Then there are the carbohydrates, which are your main energy source. Think whole grains like brown rice, quinoa, or barley. These should fill another quarter. Healthy fats, though small in portion, play a crucial role in absorbing vitamins. These can come from olive oil, avocados, or nuts. Finally, fill half your plate with a vibrant array of fruits and vegetables. They not only add color and texture but provide essential vitamins, minerals, and fiber that keep your body running smoothly. By focusing on variety, you ensure that your meals are not only nutritious but also appealing and satisfying.

Meal planning is more than just a chore—it's a powerful tool to help you make healthier choices and achieve your nutritional goals. By taking the time to plan meals ahead, you can avoid the temptation of last-minute, unhealthy food decisions that often arise from a busy lifestyle. When you're exhausted and the fridge is empty, having a planned meal ready to cook offers a quick, nutritious alternative to take-out. Planning meals also ensures your diet stays varied and balanced, helping you incorporate seasonal produce, which is fresher and often more affordable. With intentional meal planning, you can effortlessly meet your nutritional needs and enjoy diverse, exciting meals without the stress of figuring out what to eat each day.

When building balanced meals, consider using the plate method as a practical guide for portion control. This method offers a visual representation of how different food groups should be proportioned on your plate. Imagine dividing your plate into sections: half for fruits and vegetables, a quarter for proteins, and a quarter for whole grains. This simple strategy helps you maintain balance without overthinking. Another tip is to incorporate seasonal produce, which ensures a variety of nutrients and flavors in your diet. Seasonal fruits and vegetables are often fresher and more nutrient-dense, making them a healthy and flavorful addition to meals. They also tend to be more affordable and environmentally friendly, as they require less transportation and storage.

Here are a couple of meal ideas to inspire your balanced plate creations. Start with grilled chicken, seasoned to perfection, paired with fluffy quinoa. Add a hearty serving of roasted vegetables like bell peppers, zucchini, and carrots, lightly tossed in olive oil and herbs for a flavorful, nutrient-rich meal.

For a plant-based option, try a lentil salad. Mix nutrient-dense lentils with fresh greens, cherry tomatoes, cucumber slices, and a touch of red onion. Top it off with a citrus vinaigrette for a refreshing and satisfying dish packed with protein, fiber, and vibrant flavors.

Reflection Journal

Take a moment to reflect on your current meal patterns. Are there areas where you could introduce more variety or balance? Consider the foods you typically consume and envision ways to incorporate more colors and textures. Write down three changes you could make this week to create a more balanced plate. Perhaps it's trying a new vegetable, experimenting with a different grain, or simply adjusting portion sizes. Small shifts can make a big difference in your nutritional intake and overall health.

Reflection on My Current Meal Patterns Take a moment to think about the foods you typically consume. Are there areas where you notice a lack of variety or balance? How do you feel about the choices you've been making?

Introducing Variety and Balance How can you incorporate more colors, textures, and nutrients into your meals? What small shifts could enhance the overall quality of your diet?

Three Changes for This Week Write down three specific changes you'd like to make to create a more balanced plate:

Small Steps Toward Better Nutrition What small, actionable steps can you take today to start implementing these changes?

Final Thoughts How do you feel about making these adjustments? What impact do you hope these changes will have on your health and well-being?

Music Suggestion Enhance your reflection with calming and uplifting music:

- **For Peaceful Focus:** *Morning Light* by Norah Jones

- **For Creative Inspiration:** *Clair de Lune* by Debussy

- **For Motivation and Positivity:** *Here Comes the Sun* by The Beatles

Recognizing Hunger and Fullness Cues

Have you ever found yourself opening the fridge, not because you're hungry but because you're bored or stressed? Differentiating between physical and emotional hunger is key to maintaining a healthy relationship with food. Physical hunger comes on gradually, and it can be satisfied with almost any food. It's your body's way of signaling that it needs fuel. Emotional hunger, on the other hand, is sudden and often tied to specific cravings. It might lead you to reach for comfort foods that give a temporary sense of relief but leave you feeling unsatisfied. Recognizing these cues is crucial, as it allows you to respond to your body's true needs rather than its emotional desires.

Tuning into your hunger and fullness cues can transform your eating habits. When you learn to recognize satiety, you're less likely to overeat, which helps maintain a healthy weight and reduces the risk of digestive discomfort. This awareness also supports regular meal timing, preventing the cycle of extreme hunger followed by overeating. By responding to your body's natural signals, you create a balanced eating pattern that keeps your energy levels steady throughout the day. It's like listening to your internal clock, which knows when it's time to fuel up and when it's time to stop. This harmony with your body's rhythms fosters both physical and emotional well-being.

To enhance your awareness of these cues, consider keeping a hunger and fullness journal. Before and after each meal, jot down your hunger level on a scale from one to ten, with one being ravenous and ten being uncomfortably full. This practice helps you become more attuned to your body's signals, making it easier to distinguish between true hunger and other triggers. Another technique is to practice mindful breathing before meals. Take a moment to breathe deeply, tuning into your body and assessing your hunger level. This pause creates a space for reflection, allowing you to make conscious choices about what and how much to eat. These practices foster a deeper connection with your body, empowering you to eat with intention and awareness.

Real-life challenges can often blur these signals. Imagine a typical workday filled with back-to-back meetings and looming deadlines. It's easy to fall into the trap of distracted eating, where meals become an afterthought rather than a mindful act. In such scenarios, setting designated meal times can help. Even if it's just ten minutes, make sure to step away from your desk and focus solely on your meal. Emotional triggers, such as stress or anxiety, can also mask true hunger. On a stressful day, you might find yourself reaching for food as a distraction or comfort. Recognizing these patterns is the first step to addressing them. Instead of turning to food, explore alternative coping mechanisms like a quick walk or a few minutes of meditation. These practices can provide the emotional relief you're seeking without relying on food.

Reflection Journal

Take a moment to reflect on your recent meals. Consider how often you eat out of hunger versus emotion. Are there particular triggers that lead to emotional eating? Write down your observations and any patterns you notice. Identifying these triggers is the first step in addressing them, helping you cultivate a more mindful approach to eating.

Reflection on My Recent Meals Think about your recent meals. How often do you eat when you're genuinely hungry, and how often is it driven by emotions? Are there specific emotions or situations that trigger you to eat?

Identifying Emotional Eating Triggers Reflect on the moments that may have led to emotional eating. What emotions or circumstances prompt you to eat, even when you're not physically hungry?

Recognizing Patterns Are there recurring situations or feelings that influence your eating habits? How do these patterns affect your relationship with food and your overall well-being?

Small Steps Toward Mindful Eating What small actions can you take to create more awareness around emotional eating? How can you respond to emotional triggers without turning to food?

Final Thoughts How does reflecting on your emotional eating patterns make you feel? What insights have you gained, and how do you plan to approach your meals differently moving forward?

Music Suggestion Pair this exercise with calming music to help center your thoughts:

- **For Reflection and Calm:** *Weightless* by Marconi Union

- **For Clarity and Focus:** *River Flows in You* by Yiruma

- **For Grounding:** *The Sound of Silence* by Simon & Garfunkel

Savoring Food: Techniques for Slowing Down

A meal can be a moment of calm amidst the chaos of the day, offering a chance to pause and appreciate the simple pleasure of nourishment. The table is set, the aroma of freshly cooked food fills the air, and that first bite invites you to savor the flavors and textures. Savoring food is about more than just eating; it's about slowing down to fully engage with each mouthful, allowing you to enjoy the experience and enhance your connection to the food.

Slowing down also supports better digestion. Taking time to chew thoroughly helps break down food more effectively, promoting nutrient absorption and reducing the risk of bloating or discomfort. By eating mindfully, you give your body the chance to process food more efficiently, while turning a routine meal into a moment of mindfulness and enjoyment.

One effective way to slow down your eating is to put utensils down between bites. This simple action forces you to pause, giving your body time to register fullness and appreciate the meal. It might feel awkward at first, but it's a powerful tool for mindful eating. Engaging in conversation during meals is another technique. It's a natural way to pace yourself, as talking and listening prevent you from rushing through your food. By focusing on the company as well as the meal, you create a shared experience that enriches both the social and culinary aspects of dining. These methods transform eating into a leisurely activity rather than a rushed necessity, allowing you to enjoy your food and the moment fully.

The impact of savoring food goes beyond immediate satisfaction. Taking the time to enjoy your meals can significantly improve digestion. When you chew your food thoroughly, you help your digestive system do its job more effectively, breaking down nutrients and absorbing them properly. This process reduces the risk of digestive issues like bloating and discomfort, which often accompany hurried meals. Additionally, savoring food enhances your sense of fullness, allowing you to feel satisfied with less. This awareness of fullness can help prevent overeating, supporting a balanced diet and healthy weight management. By slowing down, you give your body the opportunity to communicate its needs, leading to a healthier, more enjoyable eating experience.

To practice savoring food, try engaging in mindful tasting sessions with small portions. Start with a small serving of your favorite dish, and focus on the flavors and textures as you eat. Notice the subtle nuances, the way the flavors develop, and how each bite feels. This exercise trains your senses to appreciate food more fully, enhancing your enjoyment of each meal. Another practice is mindful tea or coffee drinking rituals. Instead of gulping down your morning cup on the go, set aside a few moments to savor it. Pay attention to the aroma, the warmth of the mug in your hands, and the rich flavors as you sip. These rituals encourage you to slow down and appreciate the simple pleasures of life, turning routine tasks into moments of mindfulness.

Mindful Tasting Journal

Next time you prepare a meal, set aside a few minutes for a mindful tasting session. Serve yourself a small portion and focus on each bite. Notice the flavors, textures, and aromas. How does the food change as you chew? Take your time, putting your fork down between bites. Reflect on the experience and how it differs from eating on autopilot. By incorporating these exercises into your routine, you'll cultivate a deeper appreciation for food and a heightened sense of satisfaction from meals.

Savoring your food is an art that enriches your relationship with eating, transforming it from a necessity into a celebration of flavors and nourishment.

Reflection on My Eating Experience Next time you prepare a meal, take a moment to reflect on how you typically eat. Do you eat quickly, distracted, or mindlessly? How does that affect your overall satisfaction with the meal?

Mindful Tasting Exercise As you prepare your next meal, plan to engage in a mindful tasting session:

- **Focus on the First Bite:** Pay attention to the flavors, textures, and aromas of your food.

- **Savor Each Bite:** Take your time and notice how the food changes as you chew.

- **Pause Between Bites:** Put your fork down and breathe before taking the next bite.

Observations During Mindful Eating What did you notice about your food when you ate mindfully? Did you feel more connected to the meal? How did the experience differ from your usual eating habits?

Impact on Satisfaction and Awareness How did slowing down and being mindful of your food affect your sense of satisfaction? What new appreciation or awareness did you gain from the experience?

Small Steps to Cultivate Mindful Eating What small adjustments can you make to incorporate mindful tasting into your routine? How can you create a more intentional eating environment moving forward?

Final Thoughts How does it feel to practice mindful tasting? What benefits do you hope to experience by making it a regular habit?

Music Suggestion Pair this mindful eating experience with soothing music for relaxation and focus:

- **For Tranquil Focus:** *Sunset Lover* by Petit Biscuit
- **For Calm and Presence:** *Weightless* by Marconi Union
- **For Light and Uplifting Energy:** *Better Together* by Jack Johnson

Emotional Eating: Identifying and Overcoming Triggers

After a long day, the house is quiet, and you find yourself reaching for a bag of chips. While you're not truly hungry, the simple act of eating offers a sense of comfort, filling a need that goes beyond physical nourishment. This is the realm of emotional eating, where food becomes a response to feelings rather than hunger. Emotional eating often stems from stress, boredom, or loneliness. These emotions are powerful triggers, pushing you toward the pantry in search of solace. It's not about needing fuel; it's about filling a void or distracting from discomfort. Stress, in particular, is a common culprit. The demands of work, family, and life in general can build up, leading you to seek quick relief in the form of food. Boredom, too, can send you to the kitchen, looking for something to do or a taste to break the monotony. And when loneliness creeps in, food can feel like a friend, offering a momentary sense of connection. But this reliance on food for emotional comfort can have negative consequences, creating a cycle that's hard to break.

Emotional eating can lead to weight gain and nutritional imbalance, as the foods we reach for in these moments are often high in sugar, fat, or salt—not the most nutritious options available. This pattern can quickly spiral into a cycle of guilt and frustration. You eat to soothe emotions, then feel guilty about the choices you've made, which in turn leads to more emotional eating. It's a loop that's difficult to escape. The key to breaking free is to recognize and address the underlying emotional triggers. One strategy is to develop alternative coping mechanisms. Instead of turning to food, find other activities that offer comfort or distraction. This could be as simple as taking a walk, calling a friend, or engaging in a hobby. These activities provide a healthy outlet for emotions, helping you manage stress and boredom without relying on food. Seeking support from friends or professionals can also be invaluable. Sharing your challenges with someone who understands can offer relief and reinforce your efforts to change.

Consider real-world scenarios where emotional eating often occurs and how you might address them. Late-night snacking is a common habit, often driven by a need to unwind after a long day. To break this pattern, try creating a bedtime routine that doesn't involve food. Perhaps a warm bath or reading a book can provide the relaxation you seek. Establishing a stress-reduction plan that doesn't rely on food is crucial. This might include regular exercise, practicing mindfulness, or setting aside time each day for self-care. These practices help manage stress at its source, reducing the need to eat for emotional reasons. By identifying and addressing the triggers of emotional eating, you can build healthier habits that support both your physical and emotional well-being.

Sustainable Meal Planning and Prep

In a world that prioritizes convenience, sustainable meal planning stands out as an act of mindfulness and responsibility. It's about more than just choosing what to eat—it's about making thoughtful decisions that benefit both your health and the planet. One of the immediate benefits is the reduction of food waste and the cost savings that come with buying only what you need. This approach helps prevent spoiled produce from being thrown out, saving money and minimizing environmental impact. By focusing on seasonal, locally sourced ingredients, you not only enjoy fresher meals but also support local farmers and reduce the carbon footprint associated with transporting food long distances.

Meal prep is the practical side of sustainable planning, turning intentions into actions. Batch cooking is an excellent strategy here. By preparing large quantities of a dish and freezing portions, you ensure that you always have a healthy meal ready to go. This reduces the temptation to opt for less nutritious, quick-fix meals when time is short. Freezing meals also preserves nutrients, ensuring that you're getting the most out of your food. Another technique is utilizing leftovers creatively. Instead of letting those bits go to waste, think of them as ingredients for tomorrow's meal. Leftover roasted vegetables can become the base for a hearty soup, or extra rice can be transformed into a stir-fry. This approach not only saves food but also encourages culinary creativity, making meals more exciting and diverse.

The impact of sustainable practices on health and the environment is profound. A focus on varied diets, rich in seasonal and local produce, improves nutritional intake. You're more likely to consume a wider range of nutrients when your meals are diverse and colorful. This variety supports overall health, providing essential vitamins and minerals that your body needs to thrive. On an environmental level, these practices contribute to a lower footprint. Less waste means fewer resources are used, from the energy required to produce and transport food to the space needed to dispose of it. Every small change you make contributes to a healthier planet, creating a ripple effect that extends beyond your kitchen.

Practical tools and resources can make sustainable meal planning more accessible. Meal planning apps are a great starting point. Many offer templates that help you organize meals based on what's in your pantry, reducing unnecessary purchases. These apps often include shopping lists and recipes, streamlining the entire process. Guides to seasonal produce availability are also invaluable. They inform you about what's in season in your area, making it easier to plan meals around fresh, local ingredients. These guides not only enhance the quality of your meals but also support sustainable eating practices, aligning your diet with the natural rhythm of the seasons.

As you incorporate these sustainable practices into your routine, you'll find that they naturally lead to a more mindful and rewarding approach to food. The act of planning, prepping, and enjoying meals becomes a holistic experience, one that nourishes both body and soul. It's about creating a lifestyle that aligns with your values, one that supports your health while caring for the world around you. Sustainable eating isn't a sacrifice; it's a celebration of the abundance that nature offers, an opportunity to connect with your food in a meaningful way. As you close this chapter, reflect on the changes you can make today. Consider the impact of each meal, not just on your health, but on the planet. And as we transition to the next chapter, remember that every small step counts towards a healthier, more sustainable future.

Chapter 3

Personalized Fitness for Every Lifestyle

Imagine lacing up your sneakers, ready to begin a fitness journey that's specifically designed for your unique lifestyle. Unlike generic fitness plans, a personalized approach takes into account your individual needs, goals, and daily routines. We all have different lives—some balancing work calls with school drop-offs, others finding time for exercise during lunch breaks. This chapter will guide you in creating a fitness plan that's tailored just for you. Fitness isn't a one-size-fits-all endeavor; your journey should reflect your goals and limitations, meeting you exactly where you are.

Creating a custom fitness plan starts with a thorough self-assessment. This isn't just about your current fitness level; it's about understanding your aspirations and any hurdles you might face. Begin by reflecting on your fitness goals. Are you looking to shed a few pounds, boost your cardiovascular health, or maybe just feel more energized throughout the day? Next, assess your current fitness level. There are numerous online tools available that can help, from simple fitness tests you can do at home to more comprehensive assessments offered by local gyms or health clubs. Once you have a clear picture of your starting point and your destination, you can start setting realistic, achievable goals. Consider using a goal-setting worksheet—these are great for breaking down big ambitions into manageable steps and tracking your progress along the way.

Now that you've got your goals and current fitness level sorted, it's time to dive into the tools available to help you craft your personalized plan. The digital age offers a plethora of resources to aid in your journey. Online fitness planners are a fantastic starting point, providing structured templates that you can customize to fit your schedule. Many of these platforms allow you to input your goals and preferences, generating a plan that feels personal and achievable. Mobile apps are another invaluable resource, offering flexibility and convenience. Apps like MyFitnessPal or FitOn allow you to choose your workouts based on time, equipment, and intensity, making it easy to adapt your fitness routine as your needs evolve. These tools empower you to take control of your fitness journey, ensuring your plan grows and transforms alongside you.

To bring all these elements together, let's look at some examples of personalized fitness plans. Imagine you're a beginner focused on weight loss. Your plan might start with three days of low-impact cardio—think brisk walking or cycling—combined with two days of strength training using bodyweight exercises. Each session could be 30 minutes, fitting seamlessly into a busy schedule, with flexibility for days when life gets in the way. For someone looking to improve cardiovascular health, the plan might shift towards more aerobic exercises. Perhaps four days of moderate-intensity cardio, like swimming or jogging, paired with a weekly yoga session to enhance flexibility and reduce stress. These examples illustrate how a personalized approach can cater to diverse goals and lifestyles, transforming fitness from a chore into an integrated part of your life.

Interactive Journal: Create Your Fitness Plan

Take a moment to draft your personalized fitness plan. Begin by listing your primary fitness goals, considering both short-term and long-term ambitions. Next, assess your current fitness level using an online tool or a simple home test. With this information in hand, choose one or two online resources or apps that resonate with you. Finally, draft a weekly schedule that incorporates various exercises aligned with your goals. Remember, the key is flexibility—your plan should adapt to your life, not the other way around. This exercise is the first step in crafting a fitness journey that's uniquely yours, empowering you to take charge of your health and well-being.

Primary Fitness Goals Take a moment to reflect on your fitness journey. What are your primary fitness goals? Consider both short-term goals (e.g., improving endurance, losing weight) and long-term goals (e.g., building strength, maintaining health).

Assessing My Current Fitness Level Use an online tool or a simple home test to assess your current fitness level (e.g., endurance, strength, flexibility). Based on your findings, how would you rate your fitness today?

Online Resources or Apps What resources or apps resonate with you? How can they support your goals and provide guidance along the way?

Drafting My Weekly Fitness Schedule Create a weekly fitness plan that includes a balance of exercises. Consider strength, flexibility, endurance, and recovery. How many days a week will you work out, and what exercises will you focus on each day?

- **Monday:**

- **Tuesday:**

- **Wednesday:**

- **Thursday:**

- **Friday:**

- **Saturday:**

- **Sunday (Rest/Recovery):**

Flexibility and Adaptability How will you adjust your plan if life gets busy? What strategies will help you stay flexible while remaining consistent with your fitness journey?

Final Thoughts How do you feel about your personalized fitness plan? What steps will you take to implement it and make progress toward your goals?

Music Suggestion Pair your fitness journey with energizing music:

- **For Motivation:** *Stronger* by Kanye West

- **For Focus and Flow:** *Eye of the Tiger* by Survivor

- **For Recovery and Relaxation:** *Weightless* by Marconi Union

Time-Efficient Workouts for Busy Schedules

You've got a million things on your to-do list, and finding time for a workout can feel like just another impossible task. That's where time-efficient workouts come in, designed for those of us who need to squeeze fitness into the cracks of our day. These workouts are not just quick; they're effective, maximizing effort in a short span. High-intensity interval training (HIIT) is a powerhouse in this realm, alternating between bursts of intense activity and brief rest periods. This method not only boosts your metabolism but also keeps your heart rate up, burning calories long after you've finished. Circuit training is another gem, combining strength and cardio with minimal rest. It keeps your body guessing and your muscles engaged, offering a full-body workout in record time.

Here's an itemized approach to both routines for a more structured, guided experience:

20-Minute Full-Body HIIT Session

1. **Warm-up (3 minutes)**

    - High knees (1 minute)

    - Jumping jacks (1 minute)

    - Arm circles (1 minute)

2. **Main Circuit (12 minutes)**

    - Burpees (30 seconds)

    - Rest (30 seconds)

    - Squats (30 seconds)

    - Rest (30 seconds)

    - Push-ups (30 seconds)

    - Rest (30 seconds)

    - Mountain climbers (30 seconds)

    - Rest (30 seconds)

    - Repeat the circuit 2-3 times

3. **Cool-down (5 minutes)**
    - Forward fold stretch (1 minute)
    - Child's pose (1 minute)
    - Cat-cow stretch (1 minute)
    - Hip flexor stretch (1 minute)
    - Shoulder stretch (1 minute)

10-Minute Quick Morning Routine
1. **Warm-up (2 minutes)**
    - Jog in place (1 minute)
    - Arm swings (1 minute)

2. **Main Circuit (6 minutes)**
    - Lunges (30 seconds)
    - Plank (30 seconds)
    - Tricep dips (30 seconds, using a chair)
    - Rest (30 seconds)
    - Repeat the circuit 2 times

3. **Cool-down (2 minutes)**

    - Gentle yoga stretch (1 minute)

    - Deep breathing and side stretch (1 minute)

Both routines are designed for quick execution but still provide a full-body workout, perfect for days when you're short on time but still want to get moving!

Incorporating exercise into your workday might seem daunting, but it's more feasible than you think. Desk exercises are a brilliant way to keep moving without leaving your workspace. Consider seated leg lifts or desk push-ups during a conference call. These little bursts of activity can improve circulation and reduce stress, helping you stay focused and alert. If you're working from home, the possibilities expand. Try multitasking—walking on a treadmill while catching up on emails, or doing calf raises while waiting for your coffee to brew. These small but effective movements can add up, ensuring that exercise is a seamless part of your daily routine.

To make quick workouts even more accessible, consider leveraging technology. Fitness tracking apps like Tabata Pro or Nike Training Club offer quick workouts tailored to your preferences and goals. They provide structure, reminders, and motivation, turning your phone into a personal trainer. For those who prefer equipment, compact, multi-purpose items like resistance bands or adjustable dumbbells can transform any space into a mini gym. These tools are easy to store and versatile, allowing you to perform a variety of exercises without bulky machines. By embracing these resources, you ensure that time-efficient workouts remain engaging and effective, no matter where you are.

Interactive Journal: Quick Workout Planner

Take a moment to plan your week of time-efficient workouts. Identify three days where you can dedicate 20 minutes to exercise. Choose a combination of HIIT, circuit training, and desk exercises that appeal to you. Use a fitness app to guide your sessions, and make a list of any equipment you might need. This planner will help you visualize how fitness can fit into your schedule, empowering you to stay active, even on the busiest days.

Identifying 3 Days for Quick Workouts Look at your upcoming week and choose three days where you can dedicate 20 minutes to exercise. Mark them below:

- **Day 1:**

- **Day 2:**

- **Day 3:**

Choosing Your Workout Focus For each of the days you've selected, plan a quick workout session that includes a combination of HIIT, circuit training, and desk exercises.

Choose the one that resonates most with your goals and preferences.

- **Day 1:** (e.g., HIIT)

- **Day 2:** (e.g., Circuit Training)

- **Day 3:** (e.g., Desk Exercises)

Using a Fitness App for Guidance What app will you use to guide your sessions? List any specific workouts or programs that you'd like to follow.

Required Equipment Do you need any equipment for your quick workout sessions (e.g., resistance bands, dumbbells, yoga mat)? List any items you'll need to ensure you're fully prepared.

Visualizing Your Week of Fitness How do you feel about fitting fitness into your busy schedule? Does this plan feel achievable? How will you stay motivated to complete each session?

Final Thoughts What steps will you take to ensure you stick to your workout plan?

Music Suggestion For motivation, try these energizing tunes:

- **For High-Intensity Workouts:** *Can't Hold Us* by Macklemore & Ryan Lewis

- **For Circuit Training:** *Uptown Funk* by Mark Ronson ft. Bruno Mars

- **For Desk Exercise Focus:** *Happy* by Pharrell Williams

Functional Fitness for Everyday Life

Functional fitness is like the secret weapon you didn't know you needed. It's all about training your body to handle real-life activities with ease and confidence. Imagine moving through your day with improved mobility and stability—picking up your kids, carrying groceries, or even just climbing stairs can feel like a breeze. This approach focuses on exercises that mimic everyday movements, improving your ability to perform daily tasks safely and efficiently. By enhancing your body's natural movements, you not only reduce the risk of injury but also build a foundation of strength and resilience.

Think of squats not just as a gym exercise, but as a way to improve your leg strength for all those times you need to lift something heavy. Planks, too, are more than just a core workout; they stabilize your entire body, supporting balance and posture. These exercises are the building blocks of functional fitness, designed to make life easier and keep you moving without pain or strain. Incorporating them into your routine doesn't require fancy equipment or hours at the gym. It's about making small, consistent efforts that pay off big in your everyday life.

Integrating functional movements into your fitness plan is straightforward and incredibly rewarding. Start by combining these exercises with your existing workouts. If you're already doing strength training, add in sets of squats and planks to enhance your regimen. Functional fitness circuits are another great option, allowing you to cycle through a series of movements that target different muscle groups. These circuits can be tailored to fit your schedule, whether you have 10 minutes or half an hour. The key is consistency, ensuring these movements become second nature, seamlessly supporting your day-to-day activities.

The real magic of functional fitness lies in its practical applications. Imagine carrying a week's worth of groceries from the car to the kitchen without needing a break. Or think about how much easier it would be to bend and lift safely when tidying up your living space. These are the everyday victories that functional fitness delivers. It's about preparing your body for whatever life throws your way, ensuring you're ready to tackle tasks with strength and ease. As you build functional strength, you'll notice a newfound confidence in your movements, empowering you to live a more active and engaged life.

Functional fitness isn't just about exercise; it's about enhancing your quality of life. By focusing on movements that replicate real-world activities, you're training your body to be stronger and more resilient. This approach not only supports physical health but also boosts mental well-being, as the confidence gained from functional strength spills over into other areas of your life. Whether you're a busy parent, a dedicated professional, or an active retiree, functional fitness offers benefits that resonate across all aspects of your daily routine. Embrace these movements, and watch as they transform not only your body but also your approach to each day.

Low-Impact Exercises for All Ages

Imagine stepping into a world of movement that welcomes everyone, no matter your age or fitness level. Low-impact exercises are your gateway to a healthier lifestyle, offering a gentle yet effective way to stay active. These exercises are a boon for many reasons, starting with their reduced risk of injury. They are designed to be joint-friendly, making them ideal for those who want to keep moving without the strain that high-impact activities might cause. Whether you're recovering from an injury or simply looking for a more sustainable approach to fitness, low-impact exercises provide a safe space to move your body without fear of overdoing it. Their accessibility makes them an excellent choice for a wide range of individuals, from beginners just starting their fitness journey to seasoned athletes looking for a lighter workout.

Let's explore some of the low-impact exercises that can make a difference in your routine. Water aerobics is a wonderful option that combines resistance and support, making it perfect for those with joint concerns. The water cushions your movements, reducing stress on the joints while still providing a challenging workout. Another fantastic choice is walking. Often underestimated, walking is a powerful cardiovascular exercise that can be tailored to your pace and environment. Whether you're strolling through your neighborhood or hiking a scenic trail, walking offers numerous health benefits without the wear and tear of more intense workouts. These exercises are not only effective but also adaptable, allowing you to adjust the intensity and duration to match your needs and preferences.

Certain groups can particularly benefit from incorporating low-impact workouts into their lives. Seniors, for instance, may find these exercises crucial for maintaining mobility and independence. As we age, our bodies naturally lose some of their flexibility and strength, but regular low-impact exercise can counteract these changes, helping seniors stay active and engaged in daily activities. Beginners, too, can find solace in low-impact workouts as they ease into a new exercise routine. Starting with gentle movements allows them to build confidence and stamina, paving the way for more challenging activities down the line. These exercises create a foundation of fitness that supports long-term health and well-being, making them an essential component of any comprehensive fitness plan.

Incorporating low-impact exercises into your routine can be both simple and rewarding. Start by scheduling regular walking sessions into your week. Set aside time each day to step outside and enjoy a walk, even if it's just for ten minutes. Walking not only boosts cardiovascular health but also provides a mental reset, helping you clear your mind and reduce stress. Joining a community class or group can also enhance your experience. Many community centers offer classes like yoga or tai chi, which focus on gentle, flowing movements. These classes provide a supportive environment where you can learn and grow with others, fostering a sense of camaraderie and motivation. Additionally, consider exploring local resources such as parks or trails that encourage outdoor activities. These natural settings can inspire you to move more, turning exercise into an enjoyable part of your day.

Incorporating Yoga and Stretching for Flexibility

Imagine rolling out your yoga mat after a long day, the gentle hum of music in the background, as you start to unwind. Yoga is more than just a series of poses; it's a practice that invites you to extend beyond the limits of your physical body and into a space of mental clarity. This ancient practice opens doors to a deeper connection with yourself, promoting flexibility not only in muscles but in the mind as well. By engaging in yoga, you allow your body to stretch and strengthen, improving your range of motion and reducing the risk of injury in other activities. The beauty of yoga is that it meets you where you are, allowing you to progress at your own pace, fostering both patience and perseverance.

Stress reduction is one of yoga's most celebrated benefits. As you move through each pose, focusing on your breath and body, you enter a meditative state that calms the nervous system. This practice not only relaxes the mind but also releases physical tension stored in your muscles. Over time, regular yoga can lead to significant improvements in stress management, helping you cope with the demands of daily life with more ease and grace. One of the key elements of yoga is its ability to enhance flexibility. Through a consistent practice, you gradually increase your range of motion, enabling your body to move more freely. This increased flexibility supports everyday activities, reducing the likelihood of strains or sprains.

For those new to yoga, starting with basic poses can provide a solid foundation. Downward Dog is a staple, offering a full-body stretch that engages multiple muscle groups. This pose not only stretches your hamstrings and calves but also strengthens your arms and shoulders. Child's Pose, on the other hand, is a gentle resting position that encourages relaxation and introspection. It's a moment to pause, breathe, and reconnect with yourself amidst the bustle of life. These poses are accessible to beginners, offering a wonderful introduction to the benefits of yoga. Incorporating them into your routine can transform a hectic day into a peaceful retreat, leaving you refreshed and grounded.

Stretching, while often overlooked, plays a crucial role in maintaining a healthy body. Regular stretching prevents injuries by preparing your muscles for the demands of exercise and daily activities. Dynamic stretches, in particular, are excellent for pre-workout warm-ups, as they increase blood flow and enhance muscle elasticity. By incorporating stretches into your routine, you improve your overall performance, allowing your body to move with greater efficiency and power. Stretching also promotes better posture, reducing the risk of discomfort associated with long periods of sitting or standing. It's a simple yet effective way to support your body's health, ensuring you can enjoy an active lifestyle for years to come.

Creating a personalized stretching routine is a straightforward process. Begin by identifying areas of your body that feel tight or restricted. This awareness allows you to tailor your routine to address specific needs, enhancing its effectiveness. Incorporate stretches into your daily life, perhaps as part of your morning ritual or evening wind-down. Using props like yoga blocks or straps can enhance your stretching, providing support and deepening your practice. These tools are particularly useful for beginners, helping you maintain proper alignment and prevent injury. As you develop your routine, listen to your body, adjusting the intensity and duration of stretches based on how you feel each day. This flexibility ensures that your practice remains enjoyable and beneficial, supporting both your physical and mental well-being.

Strength Training for Beginners

Standing in front of a set of dumbbells, you might feel a mix of apprehension and excitement about the strength training ahead. It's more than just lifting weights—it's a gateway to building muscle, toning your body, and boosting your metabolism. Engaging in strength training can help you burn calories more efficiently, even when you're at rest. This happens because muscle tissue burns more calories than fat tissue, leading to a revved-up metabolism. It's like giving your body an engine upgrade, making it more efficient at burning fuel. Strength training also brings a sense of empowerment, as you witness your body becoming stronger and more capable, which can boost confidence and well-being.

Let's address some common misconceptions that might hold you back. One of the biggest myths is the fear of becoming too bulky, especially for women. The reality is, building substantial muscle mass requires specific training and dietary conditions. Most strength training routines will result in a toned physique rather than bulk. Another misunderstanding is the assumption that weight lifting is solely about aesthetics. In truth, it offers a plethora of benefits beyond appearance, such as improved bone density, better balance, and enhanced mental health. These myths can deter beginners, but understanding the real benefits can inspire you to incorporate strength training into your routine with confidence.

For those new to strength training, starting with bodyweight exercises is a fantastic way to ease into it. Exercises like push-ups and lunges are effective in building foundational strength without the need for equipment. These movements engage multiple muscle groups, improving overall fitness and coordination. As you become more comfortable, consider introducing resistance bands into your routine. They offer a versatile, portable option to add resistance and increase the challenge of your workouts. Resistance bands come in various tensions, allowing you to gradually increase intensity as your strength improves. This progression ensures that you continue to make gains without risking injury.

Proper form and technique are crucial in strength training to prevent injuries and maximize results. Each exercise has a specific form that ensures you're targeting the right muscles while protecting your joints and spine. For example, when performing a squat, you should keep your feet shoulder-width apart, engage your core, and ensure your knees don't extend beyond your toes. Maintaining these cues helps prevent strain and promotes muscle engagement. If you're uncertain about your form, consider using resources like online tutorials, fitness apps, or even a session with a personal trainer. These tools can provide guidance and feedback, helping you learn the correct techniques and build confidence in your abilities.

As you incorporate strength training into your fitness plan, remember that consistency is key. Gradually increase the intensity and complexity of your workouts as your body adapts. Listen to your body, allowing time for rest and recovery, which are just as important as the workouts themselves. By doing so, you'll create a balanced approach that supports long-term health and fitness goals. Embrace the journey of strength training with curiosity and patience, knowing that each session brings you closer to a stronger, healthier you.

Strength training is a powerful component of a well-rounded fitness routine, offering benefits that extend beyond the physical. It supports mental resilience, fosters discipline, and cultivates a sense of accomplishment. As you conclude this chapter, reflect on how the principles of personalized fitness, time-efficient workouts, functional movements, low-impact exercises, yoga, and finally, strength training, can come together to create a lifestyle that suits you. Each element plays a role in supporting your well-being, paving the way for a healthier, more vibrant life. As we transition to the next chapter, prepare to explore how these practices can be woven into daily routines, making wellness an integral part of who you are.

Chapter 4

Creating Lasting Habits

Waking up to the first light of dawn, you reach for your running shoes, not out of obligation, but because it's the best way to kickstart your day. Habits, those intricate patterns we weave into our lives, can be both our allies and our adversaries. They are the silent architects shaping our daily routines and, ultimately, our lives. Understanding how habits form is like holding the blueprint to change—we can redesign our behaviors, one brick at a time. At the heart of this transformation lies the basal ganglia, a deep-set cluster of brain structures responsible for habit memory. This region orchestrates the automatic behaviors that make up the fabric of our lives, evolving simple actions into habits through repeated practice. Habits form through a loop: a trigger prompts a routine, which leads to a reward. This cycle becomes ingrained over time, making actions second nature and freeing our minds to focus on more complex tasks.

The beauty of habits lies in their ability to grow from tiny seeds into towering oaks. The power of tiny changes, or what I like to call the 1% improvement principle, demonstrates how small, incremental adjustments can lead to profound changes over time. This concept underscores that you don't need massive leaps to make progress; instead, aim for steady, consistent growth. Imagine improving by just 1% each day. While it may seem insignificant, over the course of a year, these small changes compound, making you substantially better. This approach is less daunting than overhauling your entire routine at once, which often leads to burnout. Instead, focus on making manageable tweaks that align with your goals and lifestyle, gradually building momentum and confidence. This philosophy champions patience and persistence, reminding us that sustainable change happens over time, not overnight.

Consistency is the lifeblood of habit formation. It's the daily repetition, the showing up even when you don't feel like it, that solidifies new behaviors into habits. Like a craftsman honing their skills, it's the regular practice that refines and perfects. Missing a day isn't the end of the world, but it can disrupt the rhythm you've worked hard to establish. Think of habit building like tending to a garden; it requires consistent care and attention. Skipping a day might not ruin your progress, but it does highlight the importance of returning to your routine as soon as possible. Consistency builds trust in yourself, reinforcing the belief that you can rely on your habits to guide you through life's challenges. It's about creating a chain of positive actions, where each link strengthens the next, until your new habit feels as natural as breathing.

Aligning habits with your identity is a powerful way to strengthen your commitment. This concept, known as habit identity, suggests that when you see your habits as part of who you are, they become more deeply ingrained. Instead of saying, "I want to exercise more," shift your mindset to "I am someone who exercises regularly." This subtle change in language shifts your perception, aligning your actions with your identity. When your habits reflect your self-image, you're more likely to stick with them, as they become an expression of who you are. This alignment between habits and identity creates a sense of authenticity and purpose, motivating you to maintain your new behaviors. Consider athletes who identify as disciplined; their training becomes a natural extension of their identity, not just a means to an end. By embedding your habits into your self-concept, you create a powerful framework for lasting change.

<u>Reflection Journal</u>

Take a moment to reflect on a habit you wish to cultivate. Write down how this habit aligns with your identity and values. Consider how adopting this habit can reinforce your self-image and contribute to your personal growth. What small changes can you implement today to start aligning your actions with this new identity? Use this reflection as a guide to help you integrate your habits into the fabric of who you are, creating a path towards positive transformation.

Reflecting on a Habit I Wish to Cultivate Take a moment to think about a habit you wish to cultivate. How does this habit align with your identity and core values? Why is it important to you?

Connecting the Habit to My Self-Image How will adopting this habit help reinforce your self-image and contribute to your personal growth? What aspects of your identity does this habit reflect or support?

Small Changes to Begin the Journey What small actions or changes can you implement today or this week to start aligning your actions with your new identity? How can you make these changes feel natural and achievable?

Integrating the Habit into My Life What steps will you take to ensure this habit becomes a consistent part of your life? How will you track your progress and stay motivated?

Final Thoughts How does reflecting on this habit make you feel? What impact do you hope to see by integrating this habit into your daily routine?

Music Suggestion Pair your reflection with music that helps you focus and feel empowered:

- **For Calm and Clarity:** *Weightless* by Marconi Union

- **For Motivation and Focus:** *Rise Up* by Andra Day

- **For Positive Vibes:** *Good as Hell* by Lizzo

Habit Stacking for Seamless Integration

Ever find yourself brushing your teeth and wondering if there's a way to maximize those two minutes? That's where habit stacking comes in. It's a clever strategy that makes it easier to form new habits by linking them to existing ones. Essentially, habit stacking uses your current routines as a springboard for developing new behaviors. The idea is simple: by tacking a new habit onto an already established one, you create a sequence that feels natural and effortless. This way, the established habit acts as a trigger for the new one, making it more likely to stick.

To create a habit stack, start by identifying the daily routines that are already part of your life. These can be anything from making your morning coffee to locking the front door as you leave for work. These routines serve as anchors, providing a stable foundation for your new habits. For example, if you're looking to incorporate meditation into your day, consider adding it right after you pour your morning coffee. This way, the act of brewing coffee becomes a signal to meditate. Similarly, if you want to stretch more often, link it to brushing your teeth. As you finish brushing, use that moment to engage in a quick stretch. By associating new habits with existing ones, you sidestep the need to carve out additional time or create a new routine from scratch.

Habit stacking shines in real-world applications. Consider how you can transform your busy mornings. Perhaps you want to start expressing gratitude each day. Simply stack this new habit onto your existing routine of sitting down for breakfast. As your cereal bowl hits the table, take a moment to reflect on one thing you're thankful for. Or imagine integrating a brief workout into your evening. As soon as you change into your comfortable clothes after work, do a quick set of squats. These stacks blend seamlessly into your life, turning potential obstacles into opportunities. By piggybacking on habits you already perform, you reduce the mental load of decision-making, making it easier to adopt new behaviors.

One of the greatest benefits of habit stacking is its ability to simplify habit formation, especially for those of us juggling multiple responsibilities. By reducing decision fatigue, habit stacking streamlines your day, allowing you to focus on what truly matters. Decision fatigue occurs when you're faced with too many choices, leading to exhaustion and poor decision-making. By pre-determining when and where you'll perform a new habit, you eliminate the need for constant decision-making, freeing up mental energy. This efficiency not only makes it easier to incorporate new habits but also enhances your overall productivity and well-being.

Habit stacking is like building a chain of events, where each link is a habit that leads seamlessly into the next. This method leverages the power of routine, making new habits feel as automatic as brushing your teeth or drinking your morning coffee. Over time, these stacked habits create a ripple effect, improving various aspects of your life without overwhelming you with change. As you experiment with different habit stacks, you'll uncover a rhythm that works for you, one that aligns with your lifestyle and values. The beauty of habit stacking lies in its simplicity and adaptability, making it a versatile tool for anyone seeking to enhance their daily routine.

Overcoming Barriers to Change

We've all been there: feeling like there aren't enough hours in the day to fit in something new. One of the most common barriers to forming new habits is a lack of time. Between work, family, and personal commitments, it can seem impossible to squeeze in anything extra, even if it's beneficial. Time management becomes crucial here. Think of your schedule as a puzzle, where every piece needs to fit just right. Start by evaluating your daily routines and identifying pockets of time that can be repurposed. Perhaps it's those 15 minutes after dinner or the quiet moments before everyone else wakes up. Use these snippets wisely, turning them into opportunities for growth.

Another formidable barrier is the fear of failure. It's that little voice that whispers doubts, making you hesitate before trying something new. Yet, failure isn't the end; it's a stepping stone to learning. Reframing failure as a learning opportunity can shift your perspective. Each setback is a chance to gather insights and refine your approach. Embrace the idea that mistakes are part of the process, not a judgment of your worth. By adopting a growth mindset, you open yourself up to possibilities, seeing each attempt as progress, regardless of the outcome. This mindset encourages resilience, allowing you to bounce back stronger after each stumble.

Let's talk about environment design, a powerful yet often overlooked tool for facilitating habit change. Your surroundings influence your behavior more than you might realize. By creating physical cues for your habits, you make them more visible and accessible. For instance, if you're trying to drink more water, place a water bottle on your desk as a constant reminder. Reducing friction for positive behaviors is another effective strategy. Make the desired actions easy to start and hard to ignore. Set out your workout clothes the night before, or prep healthy snacks at eye level in the fridge. These small tweaks can significantly increase the likelihood of following through with your intentions.

On the flip side, let's address the psychological barriers that often come with change. Overcoming resistance requires mental strategies that enhance your resilience. Visualization is a powerful tool here. Picture yourself successfully adopting the new habit, feeling the emotions of accomplishment and satisfaction. This mental rehearsal primes your mind for success, making the actual process feel more natural. Self-affirmation practices can also bolster your resolve. By regularly reminding yourself of your strengths and capabilities, you build confidence in your ability to change. Write down affirmations that resonate with you and repeat them daily. They serve as a gentle nudge, encouraging you to persevere even when the going gets tough.

These strategies are your allies in the quest to overcome barriers to change. They remind you that while obstacles are real, they are not insurmountable. With a little creativity and determination, you can navigate these challenges, turning them into stepping stones on your path to personal growth and self-care.

Setting Realistic and Achievable Goals

Starting a new fitness plan or adopting healthier eating habits often begins with enthusiasm and energy. However, a common challenge arises when goals are set too ambitiously or vaguely, leading to feelings of overwhelm or uncertainty. That's where the magic of realistic goal setting comes into play. It's about crafting goals that motivate you without overwhelming, goals that are clear and achievable. This approach is crucial because it keeps you on track and builds confidence as you achieve each milestone. Enter the WISE goals framework—an approach that ensures your goals are Worthwhile, Inspiring, Specific, and Evaluated. Worthwhile means your goals should align with your values and passions, making them personally meaningful. Inspiring should spark motivation, pushing you towards action. Specific goals are clear and detailed, leaving no room for ambiguity. Lastly, goals should be Evaluated regularly, allowing you to track progress and adjust as needed. With this framework, you can create goals that not only inspire but also guide you towards success.

The process of setting goals is like mapping out a journey. It starts with defining what you want to achieve, breaking it down into manageable steps. This step-by-step approach turns a daunting task into a series of achievable actions, making progress feel natural and attainable. Let's say your goal is to improve your fitness. Begin by outlining small, specific actions, such as committing to a 15-minute walk each day. As you build confidence, gradually increase the intensity or duration of your walks. Setting timelines for accountability is another essential aspect of this process. Timelines provide structure, creating a sense of urgency that keeps you focused and motivated. Consider setting both short-term and long-term timelines, allowing you to celebrate small victories while staying committed to your larger goals. This structured approach ensures that your goals remain both realistic and within reach, paving the way for sustainable change.

Flexibility is the unsung hero of goal setting. As you pursue your goals, life happens—unexpected challenges arise or priorities shift. That's why it's essential to approach goals with a flexible mindset. Flexibility allows you to adapt and adjust your goals as needed, without feeling like you're abandoning them. It's about understanding that progress isn't always linear, and that's okay. Imagine you've set a goal to work out every morning, but suddenly, your schedule changes due to work commitments. Instead of giving up, adjust your goal to fit your new routine—perhaps working out in the evenings or finding shorter, more intense workouts. This adaptability keeps your goals relevant and achievable, even in the face of change. It encourages resilience, reminding you that setbacks are not failures but opportunities to reassess and refocus.

The beauty of setting realistic and achievable goals lies in the empowerment it brings. As you accomplish each step, your confidence grows, reinforcing your belief in your ability to achieve more. This positive reinforcement creates a cycle of success, where each achievement propels you towards the next goal. It's about building momentum, where the satisfaction of progress fuels your motivation. As you continue to refine your goals, remember to celebrate your achievements, no matter how small they may seem. Each victory is a testament to your dedication and perseverance, a reminder that you're capable of achieving great things. Whether you're striving for better health, personal growth, or professional success, setting realistic goals provides a clear path forward, guiding you closer to the life you envision.

Maintaining Motivation Through Accountability

Starting a new fitness program often begins with high spirits and enthusiasm, but as time progresses, this initial zeal can sometimes diminish, a scenario many find familiar. It's during these moments that the concept of accountability becomes indispensable, serving as a crucial bridge to sustain your commitment. Far from being just a trendy term, accountability emerges as a significant driving force that strengthens your determination to persevere. The benefits of partnering with a workout buddy or an accountability partner are profound. Such partners act as your cheerleader and motivator, applauding your achievements and providing that gentle push when your drive starts to falter. Whether it's a close friend, a family member, or a work colleague, their involvement in your fitness journey can significantly amplify your motivation. The knowledge that you have someone rooting for your success can be tremendously supportive, helping to either preserve or even elevate the enthusiasm you had at the outset.

Building accountability structures can be as simple or as elaborate as you like. Joining health and wellness groups, whether online or in your community, is a fantastic way to surround yourself with like-minded individuals who share your goals. These groups offer a sense of camaraderie and mutual motivation, turning individual efforts into a collective journey. Social media can also be a surprisingly effective tool for public commitment. By sharing your goals and progress with your online network, you create a layer of accountability that's both personal and public. The likes, comments, and encouragement you receive can be incredibly motivating, reinforcing your commitment to your goals. Plus, by putting your intentions out there, you create a sense of responsibility to follow through, knowing others are rooting for you.

Tracking progress is another cornerstone of maintaining motivation. It's one thing to set goals, but monitoring your journey provides tangible evidence of your efforts. Visual progress charts, whether digital or on paper, offer a clear view of how far you've come. They transform abstract goals into concrete achievements, providing a snapshot of your progress at a glance. This visual representation serves as a reminder that every small step counts, each effort adding to the bigger picture of success. Seeing your achievements mapped out can reignite motivation, especially on days when you might question your progress. Tracking allows you to celebrate milestones, big or small, reinforcing your dedication and propelling you forward.

The psychological impact of accountability cannot be overstated. Social reinforcement plays a crucial role in shaping behaviors, as we often adjust our actions based on the expectations and support of those around us. The knowledge that others are aware of your goals can create a sense of responsibility, motivating you to stay on track. Additionally, there's a psychological motivator that comes from the fear of disappointing others. While it's not about seeking external validation, the desire to meet the expectations of those cheering you on can be a powerful incentive. Knowing that someone else believes in your potential can bolster your own self-belief, encouraging you to push through challenges and persevere.

Accountability is about creating a support system that fosters resilience and commitment. It's the safety net that catches you when motivation wavers, offering encouragement and guidance to keep you on course. Whether it's through peer support, structured groups, or personal tracking, accountability provides a framework for success. It transforms solitary efforts into a shared experience, where each step forward is celebrated and supported. As you explore different ways to incorporate accountability into your routine, remember that it's a dynamic process, one that evolves alongside your goals and aspirations. Embrace the connections and structures that resonate with you, knowing they are allies in your pursuit of lasting change.

Tracking Progress and Celebrating Milestones

Imagine setting off on a new fitness routine or dietary change, filled with motivation and hope. As the days roll by, it's easy to lose sight of the progress you're making. This is where tracking progress becomes not just helpful but transformative. It's like looking in the mirror and seeing the subtle changes that might otherwise go unnoticed. Tracking provides a snapshot of where you started, where you are, and where you're headed. By recording daily habits, you create a log that captures each step forward. Whether it's noting the days you exercised, the meals you prepared, or the moments you practiced mindfulness, these entries serve as a tangible reflection of your efforts. Over time, analyzing trends helps you identify patterns—what works, what doesn't, and how you can fine-tune your approach for even better results.

The joy of reaching a milestone, no matter how small, is immense. Celebrating these moments is not just about the satisfaction of accomplishment, but about reinforcing your commitment and boosting your morale. It's like giving yourself a little pat on the back for a job well done. Planning small rewards for hitting these milestones can be incredibly motivating. Maybe it's a new book you've been eyeing, a relaxing spa day, or a simple afternoon off to enjoy your favorite hobby. These rewards don't have to be extravagant; they just need to be meaningful to you. Reflection on your progress to date is equally important. Taking the time to look back at what you've achieved can reignite your motivation and remind you why you started. It's about acknowledging the effort and dedication you've invested, which fuels the drive to keep going.

To effectively track your progress, consider using tools that fit seamlessly into your lifestyle. Habit tracking apps are a convenient option, offering a digital platform to log your activities and visualize your progress. These apps often come with reminders and customizable features, making it easy to stay on top of your goals. If you prefer a more tactile approach, bullet journaling techniques offer a creative and personalized way to track your journey. With a bullet journal, you can design layouts that suit your needs, incorporating habit trackers, mood logs, and reflection pages. This method allows for flexibility and creativity, turning progress tracking into a rewarding and artistic endeavor.

Reflection plays a crucial role in the development of positive habits. Regular review sessions create a space for introspection, allowing you to assess what's working and what needs adjustment. By setting aside time to reflect, you reinforce the habits you're cultivating, making them more ingrained in your daily routine. This process also highlights areas where you might need to adapt your strategies. Perhaps a certain habit isn't aligning with your schedule as well as you'd hoped, or maybe you've discovered a new approach that yields better results. Being open to change and willing to adjust your plan based on these reflections is key to long-term success.

In tracking your progress and celebrating your milestones, you create a roadmap of your journey towards holistic wellness. Each entry, each reflection, and each celebration contributes to a deeper understanding of yourself and your capabilities. As you continue to build on these habits, you're not just working towards a goal—you're transforming your lifestyle. This chapter serves as a reminder that every step, no matter how small, is a step forward. As you embrace this mindset, you'll find that the path to wellness is not about perfection but progress. In the next chapter, we'll explore how mindful living and stress management can further enhance your well-being, providing you with tools to navigate life's challenges with grace and resilience.

Chapter 5

Mindful Living and Stress Management

Stress seems to be the unwelcome guest that sneaks into your life when you least expect it. Maybe it's a looming work deadline or a tense conversation with a family member that sets your heart racing and your mind spiraling. Stress triggers are the culprits behind this all-too-familiar feeling. They are specific events or situations that provoke a stress response, and they vary widely from person to person. Identifying these triggers is crucial for managing stress effectively. By understanding what sets off your stress response, you can start to develop strategies to mitigate its impact, transforming stress from an overpowering force into a manageable part of life.

Common stress triggers often revolve around the demands of work and family. Picture this: you're juggling a pile of tasks at work, and just as you're about to make headway, an email pops up with a new deadline. Your heart rate quickens, hands get clammy, and suddenly, you're overwhelmed. Family conflicts can be another trigger, whether it's a disagreement over parenting styles or managing household responsibilities. These situations can escalate quickly, leading to a familiar knot in your stomach. Recognizing these triggers helps in understanding the physiological and emotional responses that follow. Stress isn't just in your head; it manifests physically. An increased heart rate, shallow breathing, and a flood of anxiety are telltale signs. Over time, unchecked stress can lead to chronic fatigue, weaken your immune system, and make you more susceptible to illnesses.

Identifying your unique stressors starts with self-reflection and observation. Keeping a stress diary can be an invaluable tool. Note down situations that trigger stress, your emotional and physical responses, and any patterns you notice. Over time, this journal becomes a map of your stress landscape, revealing consistent triggers and helping you anticipate them. Reflective questioning techniques can also be enlightening. Ask yourself what exactly about a situation causes stress. Is it the fear of failure, the pressure of time, or perhaps a lack of control? Understanding these nuances allows you to address the root causes, rather than just the symptoms.

Once you've identified your stress triggers, it's time to develop strategies to manage your responses. Cognitive behavioral techniques can be particularly effective. These methods encourage you to challenge and change negative thought patterns, replacing them with more balanced perspectives. For example, if a work deadline causes stress, instead of thinking, "I'll never finish," try reframing it to, "I'll tackle this one step at a time." Developing coping mechanisms is another key strategy. This might involve engaging in activities that naturally reduce stress, such as exercise, creative pursuits, or spending time in nature. These activities provide a healthy outlet for stress, allowing you to process emotions and return to a state of calm.

<u>Stress Management Journal Prompt</u>

Take a moment to write about a recent situation that triggered stress. Describe the event, your immediate reactions, and how you managed it. Reflect on what you could do differently next time. Consider how cognitive behavioral techniques could alter your perspective or how a new coping strategy might ease your response. This exercise is a step toward proactive stress management, empowering you to navigate life's challenges with resilience and clarity.

Reflecting on a Recent Stressful Situation Take a moment to write about a recent situation that triggered stress. What happened? How did you feel in the moment, and what were your immediate reactions?

How I Managed the Stress How did you manage the situation? Did you use any coping strategies or stress-relief techniques in the moment? How effective were they?

What I Could Do Differently Looking back, what could you have done differently to manage your stress more effectively? Were there any thoughts or behaviors that contributed to the stress response that you could adjust?

Incorporating Cognitive Behavioral Techniques How could cognitive behavioral techniques (such as reframing thoughts, identifying cognitive distortions, or challenging negative beliefs) help you respond differently in the future?

New Coping Strategies for Future Stress What new coping strategies could you implement the next time you encounter stress? Consider relaxation techniques, mindfulness practices, or healthier responses.

Final Thoughts How do you feel about your approach to stress management after reflecting on this situation? What will you do moving forward to build resilience and clarity in challenging moments?

Music Suggestion Pair this reflection with calming music to encourage relaxation:

- **For Relaxation and Focus:** *Weightless* by Marconi Union

- **For Stress Relief:** *Sunset Lover* by Petit Biscuit

- **For Positive Energy:** *Don't Stop Believin'* by Journey

Mindfulness Techniques for Stress Relief

Standing at the edge of a serene lake, with its calm and reflective waters, evokes a sense of stillness. Mindfulness is akin to this stillness—a tool that brings clarity and peace amidst life's turbulence. It's about focusing on the present moment, tuning into the here and now rather than getting lost in the whirlwind of past regrets or future anxieties. Mindfulness can significantly reduce stress by drawing your attention away from the chaos and back to your breath, your body, and your immediate surroundings. This practice doesn't just calm the mind; it grounds you, helping you navigate life with a steady heart and an open mind.

There are various mindfulness practices that you can explore, each offering a unique path to stress relief. One gentle and compassionate technique is Loving Kindness meditation. This practice involves silently repeating phrases of goodwill and encouragement, first directed towards yourself and then extended to others. By fostering feelings of love and connection, you cultivate a sense of peace, which can be a balm for stress. Mindful Movement is another wonderful practice. Whether it's yoga, tai chi, or simply walking, moving mindfully involves paying attention to each movement, each breath, allowing you to become fully immersed in the experience. Lastly, there's Body Scanning, where you mentally scan your body from head to toe, noticing areas of tension and relaxation, without judgment. This technique fosters a deep sense of body awareness, helping to release stress and enhance relaxation.

The benefits of regular mindfulness practice go beyond immediate stress relief. Over time, mindfulness can increase your resilience to stress, allowing you to handle life's challenges with greater ease. It helps improve emotional regulation, giving you the tools to respond thoughtfully rather than react impulsively to stressful situations. Regular mindfulness practice can also lead to enhanced concentration and emotional stability, supporting overall well-being. As you cultivate mindfulness, you may find that you're more present in your interactions, more attuned to your emotions, and more capable of maintaining balance in the face of adversity.

Starting a mindfulness practice doesn't require a major overhaul of your daily routine. It's about setting aside a few moments each day to be present with yourself. Begin by choosing a time that suits you, whether it's in the morning to set the tone for the day or in the evening to unwind. Find a quiet space where you won't be disturbed, and sit comfortably, closing your eyes if you wish. Start with a few deep breaths, allowing your mind to settle. You might choose to focus on your breathing, noting each inhale and exhale, or you might prefer a guided mindfulness resource, such as a meditation app or online video. These resources can provide structure and guidance, especially as you're starting out. Remember, mindfulness is a skill that develops over time with practice and dedication, so be patient and kind to yourself as you explore this transformative practice.

The Power of Meditation in Daily Life

Picture yourself sitting comfortably, eyes gently closed, as the chaos of the day fades into the background. This is the transformative power of meditation—a practice that not only calms the mind but also rejuvenates the spirit. Meditation serves as a powerful tool in stress management, primarily by its ability to reduce cortisol levels, the hormone that rises during stressful situations. By lowering cortisol, meditation helps alleviate stress, promoting a sense of calm and mental clarity. It's like giving your mind a much-needed rest, allowing you to approach life with renewed focus and energy.

When it comes to meditation, there's no one-size-fits-all approach. Different styles cater to various preferences, making it accessible to everyone. Transcendental meditation, for example, involves repeating a specific mantra to help settle the mind into a state of profound rest. This technique can be incredibly relaxing, providing an escape from the relentless pace of everyday life. Loving-kindness meditation, on the other hand, focuses on cultivating compassion and love towards oneself and others. It encourages you to foster positive emotions, which can have a ripple effect on your mental well-being. Guided imagery is another powerful form, where you visualize calming and peaceful scenes, helping to ease tension and promote relaxation. Each style offers unique benefits, allowing you to choose what resonates most with your needs and lifestyle.

The impact of meditation on mental health is profound. Regular practice enhances focus and concentration, sharpening your mind and enabling you to tackle tasks with greater efficiency. It's like exercising your brain, building the muscle of attention and presence. Moreover, meditation is known to improve mood, fostering positive emotions and reducing feelings of anxiety and depression. Through meditation, you create a space for self-reflection and acceptance, nurturing a healthier relationship with your thoughts and emotions. This practice empowers you to let go of negativity, embracing a more balanced and harmonious state of mind.

Incorporating meditation into your daily routine doesn't have to be a daunting task. Start by scheduling it like you would any other important appointment or class. Set aside a few minutes each day, perhaps in the morning to center yourself before the day begins, or in the evening to unwind and reflect. Consistency is key, even if it's just five minutes a day. When you find yourself overwhelmed by life's demands, take a break to meditate instead of pushing through. This pause can be incredibly refreshing, offering a moment to reset and regain composure. As you explore meditation, remember that it's a personal journey. Be patient and compassionate with yourself as you discover the style and routine that best supports your well-being.

Prioritizing Sleep for Optimal Health

Ever notice how everything feels a bit more overwhelming after a sleepless night? That's because sleep plays a crucial role in managing stress and maintaining emotional balance. When you get enough sleep, your brain has the chance to process emotions and memories, which helps regulate mood and stress levels. It's like hitting the reset button, giving your mind and body a fresh start each day. Without adequate sleep, you might find yourself more irritable and less able to cope with life's challenges. Sleep is not just about resting your body; it's about rejuvenating your mind and preparing yourself to handle whatever comes your way.

Improving your sleep quality can make a world of difference, and it starts with a consistent sleep schedule. Going to bed and waking up at the same time each day, even on weekends, helps regulate your body's internal clock, making it easier to fall asleep and wake up naturally. Creating a restful sleep environment is just as important. Think of your bedroom as a sanctuary—cool, quiet, and dark. Consider investing in blackout curtains, or use a sleep mask to keep out unwanted light. A white noise machine or fan can help drown out disruptive sounds. It's all about crafting a space that invites relaxation and supports deep, restorative sleep.

Sleep hygiene refers to the practices that promote better sleep, and it's an integral part of achieving restful nights. Limiting screen time before bed is a biggie. The blue light emitted by phones, tablets, and computers can interfere with the production of melatonin, the hormone that regulates sleep. Try to power down electronics at least an hour before bedtime. Instead, engage in relaxing activities like reading a book, taking a warm bath, or practicing gentle stretches.

These routines signal your body that it's time to wind down, easing the transition into sleep.

Restorative sleep offers a treasure trove of benefits, enhancing both physical and mental health. When you sleep well, your cognitive function improves, making it easier to concentrate, remember details, and solve problems. You might find that your mind feels sharper, and tasks that once seemed daunting become more manageable. Quality sleep also boosts your immune system. During sleep, your body produces cytokines, proteins that help fight infection and inflammation. Adequate rest gives your body the strength it needs to fend off illnesses, keeping you healthier in the long run.

Digital Detox: Reclaiming Your Mind for Mindfulness

In today's hyperconnected world, the relentless influx of notifications, emails, and social media updates can leave us feeling overwhelmed and stressed. This digital overload not only affects our mental well-being but also hampers our ability to focus and be present. A digital detox offers a refreshing pause from constant connectivity, allowing you to reclaim your time and mental space. By consciously reducing screen time, you create room for mindfulness and self-care, fostering a healthier and more intentional relationship with technology.

The Impact of Digital Overload

Constant connectivity often leads to social media comparisons and information overload, both of which contribute to heightened stress and anxiety. Scrolling through curated feeds can trigger feelings of inadequacy or FOMO (fear of missing out), while the endless barrage of news and updates can leave you feeling anxious and mentally exhausted. The pressure to keep up with this digital deluge often pulls us away from meaningful, real-world experiences.

The Benefits of a Digital Detox

Taking intentional breaks from digital devices can significantly enhance your overall well-being. Disconnecting improves sleep quality by reducing late-night disruptions from notifications and limiting the temptation to stay up scrolling. This practice supports your body's natural sleep rhythms, leading to more restful nights and energized mornings.

A digital detox also strengthens interpersonal relationships by encouraging face-to-face communication. With fewer digital distractions, you can engage more deeply with loved ones, fostering connection and understanding. By stepping away from screens, you create space for meaningful conversations, shared experiences, and genuine presence.

Practical Steps for a Digital Detox

Embarking on a digital detox doesn't mean severing ties with technology altogether. Instead, it's about finding a balance that works for you. Start by setting specific times for device use. For example, designate tech-free periods during meals or an hour before bedtime. Creating boundaries protects your mental space and encourages you to engage more fully with your surroundings.

Consider designating tech-free zones in your home, such as the dining room or bedroom, to promote device-free interactions and rest. Engage in screen-free activities to rediscover hobbies or interests that bring you joy. Whether it's reading a physical book, going for a walk, painting, or gardening, these activities enrich your life and provide opportunities for relaxation and personal growth.

Reclaiming Balance and Presence

A digital detox isn't about rejecting technology but rather about reclaiming your time and attention. By consciously choosing how and when to engage with screens, you ensure that technology serves you without overwhelming you. This mindful approach creates space for moments of presence and joy that often get lost in the digital shuffle.

Imagine starting your day without your smartphone commanding your immediate attention. Instead, you take a few moments to savor the quiet or engage in a calming morning routine. By reducing your digital consumption, you relieve the burden of being perpetually online, allowing you to refocus on the tangible world and the vibrant life unfolding around you.

Whether it's the simplicity of a conversation over coffee, the quiet beauty of a sunset, or the satisfaction of completing a creative project, these moments ground you in the here and now. A digital detox helps you rediscover these experiences, enriching your life and nurturing your mental and emotional well-being.

Cultivating a Positive Mindset

Life can sometimes feel like a relentless series of challenges, each one demanding more energy and patience than the last. In these moments, a positive mindset becomes your armor against stress. It's not about pretending everything is perfect but about finding strength in optimism. Positivity acts as a buffer, helping you bounce back from adversity. When you cultivate optimism, you're essentially building resilience, making it easier to navigate life's ups and downs. Think of it as a mental muscle that, when flexed regularly, grows stronger and more robust, ready to support you through any storm.

To foster a positive mindset, consider integrating gratitude journaling into your daily routine. This practice involves jotting down things you're thankful for, no matter how small. Perhaps it's the warmth of your morning coffee or a kind word from a friend. Focusing on gratitude shifts your perspective from scarcity to abundance, reminding you of the good that exists even on tough days. Positive affirmations are another powerful tool. These are statements you repeat to yourself, such as "I am capable" or "I am worthy." They help counteract negative self-talk, reinforcing a more constructive and encouraging dialogue in your mind. By embracing these techniques, you nurture a mindset that looks for possibilities rather than problems.

Self-compassion plays a crucial role in maintaining positivity. It's about being gentle with yourself, especially when things don't go as planned. Mindful self-reflection encourages you to observe your thoughts and feelings without judgment, allowing you to understand and accept your experiences. Practicing self-forgiveness is equally important. We all make mistakes, but dwelling on them only fuels stress. Instead, acknowledge your missteps, learn from them, and let them go. This approach reduces the emotional burden you carry, promoting a healthier, more forgiving relationship with yourself.

Maintaining a positive outlook, especially during challenging times, requires conscious effort. Surrounding yourself with positive influences is a powerful strategy. Engage with people who uplift and inspire you, whether they are friends, family, or mentors. Their energy can be contagious, helping you stay motivated and optimistic. Engaging in activities that bring joy and fulfillment is equally vital. Whether it's reading, gardening, or playing an instrument, these pursuits provide an emotional boost, reminding you of the simple pleasures in life. By actively choosing positivity, you create a mental environment where stress struggles to take hold.

As you cultivate a positive mindset and integrate these practices into your life, you'll find that stress loses some of its power. You'll feel more equipped to handle whatever comes your way, with a sense of calm and clarity. This chapter has offered tools and strategies to help you navigate stress with resilience and grace. As we move forward, you'll discover how these principles can be applied to other areas of your life, building a foundation for lasting well-being.

Chapter 6

Ethical and Environmental Considerations

Picture a grocery aisle lined with an overwhelming array of food products. Each one has a story that begins on a farm and ends on your dinner table. Understanding this journey—how food travels from farm to table—is not just about knowing what you're eating, but also about recognizing the broader impacts of your choices. The processes involved in food production and distribution are complex, often hidden behind the convenience of pre-packaged goods. Transparency in the supply chain is crucial for making informed decisions. Knowing where your food comes from allows you to consider the environmental and ethical implications of its production. Industrial agriculture, for instance, plays a significant role in this narrative. While it boosts productivity to meet global demands, it also contributes to pollution through fertilizer runoff, methane emissions, and other pollutants. This is a reminder of the unseen cost of our food choices, urging us to look beyond the labels and consider the bigger picture.

When we delve into the ethical considerations of food production, the moral issues become even clearer. Fair trade practices, for example, ensure that farmers receive fair compensation for their labor, promoting sustainable livelihoods and ethical treatment. Yet, in many agricultural sectors, labor conditions remain challenging, with workers facing long hours, low wages, and sometimes unsafe environments. These conditions highlight the need for ethical consumerism—a conscious effort to support practices that prioritize human dignity and environmental stewardship. By choosing products from ethical sources, you can drive positive change in the food industry. This concept of voting with your dollars empowers you to influence the market, encouraging companies to adopt fair and sustainable practices. Supporting local farmers is another impactful choice. By buying locally, you reduce the carbon footprint associated with long-distance transportation and contribute to the vitality of your community's economy.

Navigating the grocery store aisles, you might come across various labels and certifications indicating ethical practices. These labels can guide you in making choices that align with your values. Organic certification, for instance, assures you that the product was grown without synthetic fertilizers or pesticides, supporting biodiversity and soil health. Similarly, the Fair Trade label signals that the product was made with respect for workers' rights and environmental sustainability. These certifications serve as beacons of trust, guiding you toward products that uphold ethical standards. However, not all certifications are created equal, and understanding what each represents is key to making informed decisions. Take the time to familiarize yourself with these labels, as they provide a valuable tool in your journey toward conscientious consumerism.

Interactive Journal: Ethical Shopping Checklist

Next time you shop, use this checklist to guide your choices:

1. *Look for organic and Fair Trade certifications.*

2. *Choose products with transparent supply chains.*

3. *Support local farmers by buying from farmer's markets.*

4. *Consider the environmental impact of packaging.*

By incorporating these considerations into your shopping habits, you become part of a movement towards a more ethical and sustainable food system. This shift not only benefits the planet but also fosters a deeper connection with the food you consume, enhancing your overall well-being and supporting a *future where ethical and environmental considerations are at the forefront of our choices.*

Navigating Plant-Based Nutrition

Imagine your plate filled with vibrant colors—greens, reds, yellows—all promising not only nourishment but also a healthier planet. Plant-based diets have gained attention for their numerous benefits, and with good reason. Reducing meat consumption can significantly lower the risk of chronic diseases such as heart disease, diabetes, and certain cancers. Studies have shown that a diet rich in fruits, vegetables, whole grains, and legumes can improve overall health and longevity. But the advantages extend beyond personal health. Shifting towards plant-based eating also means a reduced carbon footprint. Meat production, particularly beef, is a major contributor to greenhouse gas emissions. By choosing more plant-based meals, you're not only taking care of your body but also making a positive impact on the environment. This dual benefit makes plant-based diets an appealing choice for those looking to live more consciously.

Transitioning to a plant-based lifestyle doesn't need to be overwhelming. Start small, and consider initiatives like Meatless Monday. This approach encourages you to dedicate just one day a week to plant-based meals, easing you into the transition. Over time, you might find yourself exploring new flavors and ingredients, broadening your culinary horizons. Another practical tip is to substitute plant proteins for meat in your favorite dishes. Think about replacing ground beef with lentils in your spaghetti sauce or using chickpeas in your salads instead of chicken. These swaps are simple yet effective, allowing you to enjoy familiar meals while incorporating more plant-based options. Gradually, these small changes can add up, leading to a more balanced and plant-focused diet.

When adopting a plant-based lifestyle, it's important to focus on key nutrients to ensure you're meeting your body's needs. Protein is often a concern for those new to plant-based diets, but there's a wide array of plant-based protein sources available. Legumes such as lentils, beans, and chickpeas are excellent choices, as are nuts, seeds, and tofu. Quinoa, a complete protein, is another versatile option. Additionally, keep an eye on vitamin B12, a nutrient primarily found in animal products. B12 is crucial for nerve function and red blood cell production, so consider supplementation or fortified foods to maintain adequate levels. By paying attention to these nutrients, you can maintain a balanced and healthy diet while embracing a plant-based lifestyle.

Misconceptions about plant-based nutrition can sometimes deter people from making the switch. One common myth is that plant-based diets are protein-deficient. However, a varied diet that includes a range of plant-based proteins can easily meet your protein needs. It's all about balance and diversity, ensuring that your meals include a mix of legumes, grains, vegetables, and other protein-rich foods. Another misconception is that plant-based eating is bland or restrictive. In reality, it's an opportunity to experiment with new recipes and flavors, transforming simple ingredients into delicious and satisfying meals. By debunking these myths, you can approach plant-based nutrition with confidence and creativity.

Embracing plant-based nutrition is a journey of discovery, both for your palate and your well-being. As you explore the possibilities, you'll find that plant-based eating is not only healthful but also deeply satisfying. It encourages you to engage with your food, experimenting with textures and flavors that might have been previously overlooked. This approach fosters a mindful relationship with eating, aligning with a holistic lifestyle that values self-care and sustainability. Each plant-based meal is a step toward a healthier you and a healthier planet, creating a ripple effect of positive change.

Balancing Ethical Eating with Personal Health

Navigating the intersection of ethical eating and personal health can sometimes feel like a tightrope walk. On one hand, you want to make choices that reflect your values, like reducing your carbon footprint or supporting fair labor practices. On the other hand, your body has nutritional needs that must be met for you to thrive. This balance can seem daunting, especially if you have personal dietary restrictions, such as allergies or intolerances, that further complicate your choices. The key is to prioritize a balanced diet that provides all the nutrients you need while still honoring your ethical commitments. It's about creating a diet that satisfies both your conscience and your body's requirements.

One approach to achieving this balance is embracing a flexitarian lifestyle, which focuses on reducing meat consumption without eliminating it entirely. This diet allows for flexibility, letting you enjoy plant-based meals most of the time while still partaking in your favorite non-plant dishes. By incorporating diverse food sources, like legumes, grains, and vegetables, you can ensure that your diet is rich in essential nutrients. This variety not only meets your nutritional needs but also supports ethical eating by reducing reliance on resource-intensive animal products. The flexitarian approach is particularly suitable for those who want to make a difference without committing to a fully plant-based lifestyle.

Moderation plays a crucial role in maintaining this balance. It's about acknowledging that occasional indulgences are part of life and don't have to derail your ethical eating goals. Allow yourself to enjoy a non-ethical choice now and then, whether it's a special occasion or a craving you can't shake. The key is to keep these indulgences rare and mindful, ensuring they don't become the norm. By practicing moderation, you can enjoy the foods you love without compromising your ethical values or your health. It's a realistic approach that lets you savor life's pleasures while staying grounded in your principles.

Consider the Mediterranean diet, often hailed as a model of balanced and ethical eating. It emphasizes whole foods, like fruits, vegetables, whole grains, and healthy fats, while incorporating sustainably sourced fish and poultry. This diet highlights the importance of quality over quantity, focusing on fresh, local, and seasonal ingredients that support both health and the environment. Similarly, a plant-forward omnivorous diet allows for a flexible approach, prioritizing plant-based meals while occasionally including ethically sourced animal products. These diets serve as examples of how you can enjoy diverse, satisfying meals that align with both ethical and health-conscious goals.

Balancing ethical eating with personal health is a dynamic process, requiring you to adapt and adjust as needed. It encourages you to be mindful of your choices, both for your health and for the planet. By exploring various dietary options and experimenting with new foods, you can find a balance that's uniquely yours. This balance is not about perfection but about progress, making small, meaningful changes that reflect your values and priorities. As you navigate this path, remember that every choice counts and contributes to a healthier you and a more sustainable world.

Reducing Food Waste: Practical Tips

Imagine you're preparing dinner, chopping vibrant vegetables and arranging them on your counter. But before you know it, you realize that the fridge is filled with forgotten leftovers and expired produce. This is a common scenario, and it contributes significantly to food waste, which has profound environmental consequences. When food ends up in a landfill, it decomposes and releases methane—a potent greenhouse gas—into the atmosphere. This process makes food waste a major contributor to climate change. Moreover, the resources used to produce this wasted food—water, energy, and labor—are also squandered. Think about the energy it takes to grow, harvest, transport, and store food that is ultimately discarded. This wastefulness strains our planet's finite resources and emphasizes the need for change.

At home, there are practical strategies you can adopt to minimize food waste. Meal planning is a simple yet effective method. By planning your meals for the week, you can create a shopping list that ensures you only buy what you need. This approach prevents over-purchasing and reduces the likelihood of food going bad before you can use it. Alongside meal planning, proper storage techniques play a vital role in extending the freshness of your food. For instance, storing fruits and vegetables in the right humidity settings in your fridge can significantly prolong their shelf life. Airtight containers for grains and cereals help maintain their quality, keeping them fresh and ready for use.

Leftovers, often seen as a burden, can actually be an opportunity for culinary creativity. Instead of letting them languish in the back of the fridge, consider how they can be transformed into new meals. Last night's roasted chicken, for example, can become today's chicken salad or tomorrow's hearty soup. By thinking creatively, you can turn leftovers into exciting dishes that save both time and money. Composting is another effective strategy for reducing food waste. By composting food scraps, you can divert waste from landfills and create nutrient-rich soil for gardening. This process not only reduces methane emissions but also enriches the soil, supporting a more sustainable ecosystem.

Community initiatives can amplify these efforts, making a significant impact on food waste reduction. Food sharing networks, for instance, connect individuals with surplus food to those in need, ensuring that excess food finds a home instead of a landfill. These networks promote a sense of community and generosity, transforming potential waste into valuable resources. Supporting food recovery programs is another way to contribute. These programs work with local businesses and organizations to redistribute surplus food to charities and food banks. By participating in or supporting these initiatives, you play a part in creating a more sustainable and equitable food system.

Interactive Journal: Food Waste Reduction Challenge

For one week, challenge yourself to reduce food waste at home. Here's how:

1. Plan your meals and stick to your shopping list.

2. Organize your fridge to ensure older items are used first.

3. Get creative with leftovers, making them into new meals.

4. Start a compost bin for food scraps.

By actively engaging in these practices, you not only minimize waste but also develop a deeper appreciation for the food you consume. Each small action contributes to a larger movement towards sustainability, proving that individual efforts can lead to collective change.

Reflection on My Eating Experience Next time you prepare a meal, take a moment to reflect on how you typically eat. Do you eat quickly, distracted, or mindlessly? How does that affect your overall satisfaction with the meal?

Mindful Tasting Exercise As you prepare your next meal, plan to engage in a mindful tasting session:

1. **Focus on the First Bite:** Pay attention to the flavors, textures, and aromas of your food.

2. **Savor Each Bite:** Take your time and notice how the food changes as you chew.

3. **Pause Between Bites:** Put your fork down and breathe before taking the next bite.

Observations During Mindful Eating What did you notice about your food when you ate mindfully? Did you feel more connected to the meal? How did the experience differ from your usual eating habits?

Impact on Satisfaction and Awareness How did slowing down and being mindful of your food affect your sense of satisfaction? What new appreciation or awareness did you gain from the experience?

Small Steps to Cultivate Mindful Eating What small adjustments can you make to incorporate mindful tasting into your routine? How can you create a more intentional eating environment moving forward?

Final Thoughts How does it feel to practice mindful tasting? What benefits do you hope to experience by making it a regular habit?

Music Suggestions Pair this mindful eating experience with soothing music for relaxation and focus:

- **For Tranquil Focus:** *Sunset Lover* by Petit Biscuit

- **For Calm and Presence:** *Weightless* by Marconi Union

- **For Light and Uplifting Energy:** *Better Together* by Jack Johnson

Sustainable Sourcing: Making Informed Choices

Imagine standing in your local market, surrounded by an array of vibrant produce. Each item represents more than just food; it embodies a choice that impacts both your health and the planet's future. Sustainable sourcing is about those choices. It involves obtaining ingredients in a way that maintains the long-term viability of food systems and preserves biodiversity. This approach ensures that the land, waters, and ecosystems used in food production remain healthy for future generations. By prioritizing sustainability, we can support practices that protect natural resources and promote ecological balance. This way, the food we enjoy today doesn't compromise the ability of future generations to enjoy the same.

Identifying sustainably sourced products can feel daunting, but there are tools to guide you. Eco-labels and certifications provide insight into the practices behind your food. Certifications like Rainforest Alliance and Marine Stewardship Council ensure that products are produced with minimal environmental impact, promoting ethical and sustainable farming methods. Transparency and accountability are crucial, too. Brands that openly share their sourcing practices and maintain traceable supply chains offer reassurance about the sustainability of their products. By seeking out these labels and supporting brands that prioritize sustainability, you can make informed choices that align with your values and contribute to a healthier planet.

Consumer demand plays a pivotal role in promoting sustainability. As consumers, we have the power to drive market change through our purchasing decisions. When we support brands that embrace sustainable practices, we send a clear message about the importance of environmental responsibility. This demand encourages more companies to adopt sustainable sourcing, creating a ripple effect that can transform entire industries. Whether it's choosing a company that prioritizes ethical labor practices or one that focuses on reducing carbon emissions, your choices matter. They can inspire widespread adoption of sustainable practices, benefiting both the environment and the communities involved in food production.

Consider the success stories of sustainable sourcing practices that have made a significant impact. Community-supported agriculture programs connect consumers directly with local farmers, providing access to fresh, seasonal produce while supporting small-scale, sustainable farming. These programs reduce the distance food travels, minimizing its carbon footprint and fostering local economic growth. Another example is sustainable seafood sourcing, which focuses on harvesting fish in ways that maintain healthy populations and ecosystems. Initiatives like these demonstrate how sustainable sourcing can create positive change, benefiting both the environment and those who rely on it for their livelihoods. By participating in such programs, you contribute to a movement that supports sustainability and promotes responsible stewardship of natural resources.

The Environmental Impact of Dietary Choices

When you think about what you eat, it's easy to focus just on taste and nutrition. But your meal choices also play a crucial role in shaping the environment. Different diets come with varying ecological footprints. For instance, plant-based diets typically have a smaller environmental impact compared to meat-heavy diets. This is largely because producing meat, especially beef, involves significant resources like water and land, resulting in high greenhouse gas emissions.

In contrast, plant-based foods require fewer resources and produce less pollution, making them a more sustainable choice. Yet, it's not just about meat vs. plants. Monoculture crops, such as corn and soy, often used to feed livestock, can also harm the environment. They contribute to soil degradation and biodiversity loss, creating a complex web of environmental challenges tied to our food choices. Understanding these impacts helps you make informed decisions, not just for your health, but for the planet.

There are practical strategies you can adopt to reduce the environmental impact of your diet. One effective approach is to prioritize local and seasonal foods. These options are often fresher and require less energy for transportation and storage. By choosing what's in season, you also support local farmers and reduce the carbon footprint of your meals. Additionally, cutting back on processed foods is beneficial. Processing often involves extra energy and resources, not to mention packaging that can end up in landfills. Instead, focus on whole foods that are closer to their natural state. They not only have a lower environmental impact but also offer better nutrition. Making these simple changes can have a significant positive effect on the environment.

Considering the carbon-conscious aspect of your diet can further guide your choices. A carbon-conscious diet focuses on reducing the carbon footprint of your meals. You can start by calculating the carbon impact of the foods you eat. There are various online tools and resources that can help you understand which foods have higher carbon emissions and why. Once you have this knowledge, you can plan low-carbon meals, emphasizing foods with lower emissions. This might mean more plant-based dishes or incorporating sustainably sourced fish and poultry. It's about making thoughtful choices that align with sustainability goals. By being mindful of the carbon footprint of your diet, you contribute to a healthier planet.

To put these ideas into practice, consider engaging in environmentally conscious dietary habits. Participating in community gardens is a great way to access fresh, local produce while reducing reliance on commercially grown foods. These gardens foster community spirit and offer opportunities to learn about sustainable agriculture. Another impactful practice is supporting regenerative agriculture. This method focuses on regenerating soil health and enhancing ecosystem biodiversity. By choosing products from farms that use regenerative practices, you support a system that prioritizes long-term environmental health. These practices remind us that our food choices extend beyond our plates, influencing the world around us in profound ways.

As we wrap up this chapter, it's clear that our dietary choices are deeply intertwined with environmental health. From reducing carbon footprints to supporting sustainable farming, what we eat matters not just for our bodies but for the planet. Embracing eco-friendly habits is part of a broader commitment to wellness, one that considers both personal health and global impact. With these insights, you're equipped to make choices that reflect a holistic approach to well-being, leading seamlessly into our next chapter on interactive journaling for self-discovery.

Chapter 7

Interactive Journaling for Self-Discovery

Imagine for a moment that you're in a bustling café, a steaming cup of coffee beside you, and a journal open in front of you. It's not just a blank page; it's a canvas for your thoughts, a place where your inner world meets the outer one. Journaling is more than just jotting down events of the day. It's a tool for understanding yourself, a way to sift through the noise and distill your experiences into something meaningful. In our fast-paced lives, where everything demands our attention, taking a moment to write can feel like a breath of fresh air, a pause that allows you to reflect and recalibrate.

Reflective journaling is a process where you pour your thoughts and emotions onto paper, clarifying them in the process. It acts as a mirror, allowing you to see your thoughts more clearly and develop a deeper understanding of your feelings. By consistently journaling, you enhance your self-awareness, recognizing patterns and triggers in your behavior that might otherwise go unnoticed. This practice encourages introspection, helping you make sense of complex emotions and experiences. In doing so, you gain insight into yourself, fostering a greater sense of self-acceptance and understanding.

The mental health benefits of journaling are well-documented. Regular journaling can reduce stress and anxiety by providing a safe outlet for expressing emotions. When you write about your fears, worries, or frustrations, you externalize them, reducing their power over you. This act of expression can lead to improved mood and emotional regulation, helping you navigate life's challenges with more resilience. Studies have shown that expressive writing can lower blood pressure, improve lung and liver function, and even reduce depressive symptoms. By incorporating journaling into your routine, you create a space for emotional release and healing, promoting overall well-being and mental clarity.

Supporting the benefits of journaling, research has demonstrated its therapeutic potency. Engaging in expressive writing can significantly reduce depressive symptoms, enhance mood, and contribute to better overall physical health. This approach, free from medication, is increasingly being incorporated into psychotherapy to assist in the management of anxiety, depression, and stress. Journaling fosters a welcoming space for mental experiences, aiding in psychological well-being and therapeutic success. The act of recording one's thoughts and emotions initiates a journey of introspection and growth, leading to a healthier mind and a more understood self. The advantages of keeping a journal go far beyond providing temporary solace, opening doors to lasting self-discovery and deeper comprehension.

There are various styles of journaling you can explore, each offering its own unique benefits. Free-writing, for instance, is a stream-of-consciousness approach where you let your thoughts flow without worrying about structure or grammar. This method allows you to tap into your subconscious, uncovering insights that might be hidden beneath the surface. It's about unfiltered expression, capturing the essence of your thoughts and emotions as they arise. On the other hand, structured journaling involves using prompts to guide your writing. These prompts can help focus your reflections, encouraging you to delve into specific themes or aspects of your life. By providing a framework, structured journaling allows you to explore your thoughts more deeply, fostering greater clarity and understanding.

Interactive Exercise: Journaling Starter Prompts

Set aside 10 minutes each day to explore your thoughts through journaling. Start with these prompts: "What is one thing I learned about myself today?" and "What emotions did I experience, and why?" Try both free-writing and structured approaches to discover what resonates with you. This practice is not about perfection; it's about creating a dialogue with yourself, a conversation that unfolds on the page. As you engage with these prompts, allow yourself to be curious and open, letting your insights guide you toward greater self-awareness and personal growth.

Reflection on My Nutrition Tracking Take a moment to reflect on your current approach to nutrition. Do you find yourself guessing what's in your meals, or do you have a system in place? How do you track your food, if at all? How accurate or helpful do you find your current method?

What's Working Well Write down what you think works well in your current nutrition tracking. Are there any habits or tools that help you make healthier food choices?

Areas to Improve Reflect on areas where you feel your tracking could improve. Do you miss meals or forget to log certain items? Are there any gaps that leave you unsure about your nutrient intake?

The Role of Digital Tools Consider how a digital tool could support your goals. Would it help with meal planning, nutrient tracking, or accountability? How might an app streamline your process and make tracking easier?

Choosing the Right App Identify any needs or features that you would like a nutrition app to have. Would you prefer one with barcode scanning, meal suggestions, or nutrient breakdowns?

Small Steps to Improve Tracking What small steps can you take today to improve your nutrition tracking? Could you try a new app or make a habit of tracking after each meal?

Final Thoughts How does tracking your nutrition make you feel? What do you hope to achieve with a more structured approach to tracking your meals?

Music Suggestions Pair this reflection with soothing or motivational music for focus:

- *For Focus and Calm*: *Weightless* by Marconi Union
- *For Motivation and Clarity*: *Good Life* by OneRepublic

- *For Relaxation*: *Sunset Lover* by Petit Biscuit

This journaling practice allows you to slow down, reflect, and gain insights that support your personal growth and mindfulness journey.

Journaling Prompts for Mindful Eating

Picture yourself at the dinner table, plate full of vibrant colors, each bite a sensory delight. Yet, how often do we really tune into the experience of eating? Journaling can transform this everyday act into a mindful practice, helping you become more aware of your eating habits and patterns. It's not just about what you eat, but how and why. By journaling, you can uncover emotional triggers that prompt you to reach for food, whether it's stress, boredom, or even joy. This awareness is crucial, as it allows you to reflect on your eating experiences, helping you distinguish between physical hunger and emotional cravings. Writing about these moments can reveal patterns you might not have noticed, fostering a healthier relationship with food.

To guide you on this path, consider using specific prompts to explore your relationship with eating. Start by asking, "What emotions do I feel before, during, and after eating?" This question encourages you to pause and assess your emotional state, offering insights into your motivations for eating. Another powerful prompt is, "How does my body feel after each meal?" Reflecting on your body's physical responses can help you understand the effects of different foods, promoting better choices in the future. These prompts serve as gentle guides, leading you to deeper insights into your eating habits. They encourage you to slow down and engage with your meals, turning eating into a mindful practice rather than a hurried task.

Using prompts can be incredibly beneficial, offering a structured way to engage with your thoughts and feelings around food. They act as anchors, focusing your reflections and helping you uncover the "why" behind your eating habits. This practice can lead to mindful eating, where you savor each bite and listen to your body's hunger cues. By regularly engaging with these prompts, you develop a habit of mindfulness that extends beyond mealtimes, influencing your approach to food and health. The insights gained through journaling can empower you to make conscious choices, fostering a balanced and intuitive way of eating.

Integrating journaling into your mealtime routine doesn't have to be complicated. Consider starting with a pre-meal reflection exercise. Before you begin eating, take a moment to jot down your hunger level and emotional state. Are you truly hungry, or are you eating for another reason? This simple practice can ground you in the present moment, aligning your eating with your body's needs. After your meal, engage in a post-meal journaling session. Reflect on how the meal made you feel, both physically and emotionally. Did it satisfy your hunger? Did it bring you joy or comfort? By dedicating a few minutes to these reflections, you create a mindful space that enhances your connection to food.

Transforming your eating habits through journaling is a journey of self-discovery. It's about cultivating a deeper understanding of what drives your food choices and how they affect your well-being. By incorporating these practices into your daily routine, you foster a sense of mindfulness that extends to all areas of your life. Each meal becomes an opportunity to explore and learn, guiding you toward a more intuitive and balanced approach to eating. As you continue to engage with these prompts, you'll find that they not only enhance your relationship with food but also support your overall health and happiness.

Tracking Emotional Well-Being

Picture your emotions as waves, constantly shifting and changing, sometimes calm and sometimes tumultuous. Keeping track of these emotional tides through an emotional well-being journal can be a powerful tool for understanding your mental health. By doing so, you gain insights into your patterns and mood fluctuations, recognizing what triggers certain emotional responses. This awareness becomes invaluable, allowing you to anticipate how you might feel in different scenarios and prepare accordingly. Think of it as a map that charts your emotional landscape, guiding you through the peaks and valleys that we all experience in life.

To effectively track your emotional states, consider incorporating daily mood charts into your routine. These visual tools allow you to record your feelings on a scale—maybe from one to ten—giving you a clear picture of how your emotions ebb and flow over time. Another useful technique is the emotion wheel, a colorful chart that helps identify and expand on basic feelings like happiness, anger, or sadness, encouraging you to explore the nuances of your emotions. By labeling your feelings more precisely, you begin to understand the complexity of your emotional experiences, which can lead to greater clarity and acceptance of your mental states.

Understanding emotional patterns through tracking can significantly enhance your well-being. As you become more attuned to your emotional rhythms, you learn to anticipate and manage your responses more effectively. This anticipation allows you to prepare for challenging situations, equipping you with strategies to cope when emotions run high. Moreover, tracking emotions increases your emotional intelligence, helping you recognize not just your feelings but also the emotions of those around you. This awareness can improve your relationships, as you become more empathetic and understanding in your interactions with others.

To support your emotional journaling practice, explore various tools and resources that cater to different preferences and lifestyles. Mood tracking apps, for instance, are convenient options for those who prefer digital solutions. Apps like MoodPath or Daylio offer features that allow you to log your emotions throughout the day, often including prompts or questions to guide your reflections. For those who enjoy a more tactile approach, bullet journaling templates for emotions provide a structured yet customizable layout for recording your feelings. These templates can be tailored to your needs, offering a creative outlet that encourages regular engagement with your emotional tracking practice.

Consider incorporating an interactive element, such as a checklist to help establish your emotional tracking routine. Begin by selecting a method that resonates with you, whether it's a digital app or a paper journal. Commit to logging your emotions at least once a day, perhaps at a consistent time like morning or evening. Use your mood tracker to note any patterns, triggers, or significant events that influence your emotional state. Over time, reflect on the data you've gathered to identify recurring themes or insights. This checklist serves as a guide to ensure that your emotional tracking becomes a habit, supporting your journey toward greater self-awareness and emotional balance.

Visualizing Your Health Goals

Picture yourself standing on a mountaintop, the wind in your hair, and a clear vision of where you want to be in your wellness journey. Visualization is a powerful tool that can transform your goals from distant dreams into tangible realities. By clearly imagining your desired outcomes, you create a mental blueprint that guides your actions and decisions. This process isn't just about daydreaming—it's about harnessing the mind's ability to influence your motivation and clarity. Visualization connects your intentions with your achievements, making your goals feel more attainable and less abstract. When you visualize success, you're not just hoping for it; you're actively preparing your mind to recognize opportunities and overcome obstacles. This practice instills a sense of confidence, reinforcing your commitment to your health goals and helping you stay focused on what truly matters.

To bring your visions to life, consider using techniques that create a vivid mental picture of your desired outcomes. Vision boards are a popular method, where you gather images and words that represent your health and wellness aspirations. These boards serve as a visual reminder, keeping your goals at the forefront of your mind. Whether it's a picture of a serene yoga pose or a quote about resilience, each element on your board should resonate with your personal journey. Guided visualization exercises are another effective approach, where you close your eyes and immerse yourself in a detailed mental scenario of achieving your goals. Imagine the sights, sounds, and emotions associated with reaching your desired state of health. By engaging your senses, you make the experience more real, enhancing your motivation to work towards it.

The benefits of goal visualization are profound, as this practice can significantly reinforce your commitment and focus. When you regularly visualize your goals, you create a mental rehearsal that prepares you for success. This rehearsal boosts your confidence, as your mind becomes accustomed to the idea of achieving what you set out to do. The vivid imagery associated with visualization can reignite your motivation during times of doubt or challenge. It reminds you of the reasons behind your efforts, helping you push through obstacles with renewed determination. Visualization transforms your aspirations from mere wishes into actionable plans, solidifying your resolve to pursue them with dedication and passion.

To make visualization a regular part of your routine, incorporate practical exercises that align with your goals. Creating a collage of health aspirations is a creative way to engage with your vision. Gather magazines, printouts, or even your own drawings that symbolize your wellness dreams, and arrange them on a board or in a journal. This tactile activity encourages reflection and reinforces your goals each time you see it. Another exercise involves daily affirmation practices related to your goals. Start each day with positive statements that affirm your commitment to your health journey. Whether spoken aloud or written down, these affirmations serve as a reminder of your intentions and encourage a mindset of positivity and possibility.

Visualization is more than a practice—it's a mindset that empowers you to take charge of your health and well-being. By vividly picturing your goals, you create a mental landscape where success feels not only possible but inevitable. This mindset fosters resilience, motivating you to navigate challenges with grace and determination. As you continue to engage with visualization, you'll find that it enhances your ability to stay focused, inspired, and aligned with your aspirations. Each visualization session strengthens your belief in yourself and your capacity to achieve the outcomes you desire. With this powerful tool at your disposal, you're equipped to transform your health goals into a fulfilling reality.

Gratitude Practices for Positivity

Imagine waking up and, instead of diving headfirst into the day's to-do list, you take a moment to acknowledge what you're grateful for. This small shift in focus can transform your entire outlook. Gratitude is a powerful tool that can help shift your attention from what's lacking in life to the abundance you already have. By practicing gratitude, you develop a positive mindset that reduces negative thinking patterns. It's like training your brain to see the glass as half full, focusing on the silver linings rather than the clouds. Gratitude encourages you to pause and appreciate the good, even amidst stress or uncertainty. This shift in perspective can lead to a more optimistic and contented life.

One effective way to cultivate gratitude is through regular journaling exercises. Start by writing down three things you're grateful for each day. These don't have to be grand gestures; they can be as simple as a warm cup of coffee, a smile from a stranger, or a moment of peace in your hectic schedule. By recording these moments, you create a tangible record of positivity that you can revisit whenever you need a boost. Reflecting on positive interactions with others is another powerful exercise. Think about a recent conversation that uplifted you or an act of kindness you received. Write about how it made you feel and why it mattered to you. These reflections not only enhance your appreciation for the present but also strengthen your connections with those around you.

The benefits of gratitude extend far beyond the journal page. Practicing gratitude can enhance emotional resilience, helping you bounce back from setbacks with greater ease.

When you focus on the positive, you cultivate a mindset of abundance, which can improve your relational well-being. You become more empathetic and understanding, as gratitude encourages you to see the good in people and situations. This shift in perspective can lead to stronger, more fulfilling relationships, as you approach interactions with kindness and appreciation. Gratitude also fosters a sense of contentment, reducing the tendency to compare yourself to others and increasing satisfaction with your own life.

Integrating gratitude into your daily life doesn't have to be a daunting task. Consider starting a gratitude journal that you write in before bed. This simple practice allows you to end the day on a positive note, reflecting on the good things that happened and setting the stage for a restful night's sleep. Sharing gratitude with friends or family is another wonderful way to make it a habit. Perhaps over dinner, you each share one thing you're thankful for, turning gratitude into a shared experience. This practice not only strengthens your relationships but also creates a supportive environment where positivity is celebrated and encouraged.

As you incorporate these gratitude practices into your routine, you'll likely notice a shift in how you perceive and interact with the world. The more you focus on the positive aspects of life, the more they'll multiply, creating a cycle of joy and appreciation. Gratitude becomes a lens through which you view your experiences, transforming challenges into opportunities for growth and connection. This practice is not about ignoring difficulties but rather about finding the good amidst the chaos. By embracing gratitude, you open yourself up to a world of positivity and possibility, enriching your life in ways you may not have imagined.

Creating a Personalized Wellness Journal

Imagine your wellness journal as a trusted companion on your path to health. It's not just a collection of pages; it's a personalized space that reflects your unique journey, goals, and values. By customizing your journal, you create a tailored guide that aligns with your aspirations and needs. This personalization is key, as it ensures that every entry, every thought, and every plan resonates with who you are and what you aim to achieve. Your journal becomes a reflection of your personal wellness narrative, capturing the essence of your journey toward holistic health.

Setting up your wellness journal involves thoughtful design and organization, turning it into a tool that supports your growth. Start by selecting sections for different aspects of wellness that matter to you, such as nutrition, exercise, mental health, and personal growth. Each section offers a dedicated space to explore and document your progress, creating a comprehensive overview of your wellness journey. Incorporate inspirational quotes or images that resonate with your goals, infusing your journal with motivation and positivity. These visual elements serve as daily reminders of your aspirations, encouraging you to stay focused and inspired. By organizing your journal in this way, you create a tool that not only supports your wellness goals but also inspires and uplifts you along the way.

The power of a personalized journal lies in its ability to enhance motivation and engagement, offering a sense of ownership and accountability. When your journal aligns with your personal wellness goals, it becomes a source of inspiration, guiding you toward meaningful change. The customization process encourages you to take ownership of your journey, fostering a deeper connection with your goals. This alignment increases accountability, as the journal becomes a tangible representation of your commitment to health and well-being. By regularly engaging with your personalized journal, you maintain momentum and focus, propelling you forward on your path to holistic health.

Consider exploring creative journal layouts that make your wellness journey engaging and functional. Monthly goal-setting pages can help you outline your aspirations and track your progress, providing a clear roadmap for your wellness journey. These pages offer a space to set intentions, reflect on achievements, and adjust your goals as needed. Wellness trackers for habits and progress are another valuable addition, allowing you to monitor behaviors and celebrate milestones. These trackers provide visual feedback on your efforts, reinforcing positive habits and motivating you to continue. By incorporating these elements into your journal, you create a dynamic and interactive tool that supports your wellness journey in a meaningful way.

As you continue to engage with your personalized wellness journal, you'll discover its capacity to transform your approach to health and well-being. The journal becomes a living document that evolves with you, capturing your growth and achievements. It serves as a reminder of your resilience, adaptability, and dedication to personal growth. This journey of self-discovery and wellness is not just about reaching a destination; it's about embracing the process and finding joy in each step. A personalized journal is more than a record of your journey; it's a celebration of your commitment to living a balanced and fulfilling life.

Your personalized wellness journal is a powerful tool that supports your journey toward holistic health. By customizing its design and incorporating elements that resonate with you, you create a journal that reflects your unique path. This personalization enhances motivation and engagement, aligning the journal with your wellness goals and fostering accountability. As you explore creative layouts and track your progress, you'll find that your journal becomes an invaluable companion on your journey to health and well-being. It captures your growth, celebrates your achievements, and inspires you to continue moving forward with confidence and determination.

Chapter 8

Enhancing Your Wellness Journey with Technology

Think back to the last time you felt the rush of excitement when starting something new—a new project, hobby, or perhaps a fitness routine. That initial burst of motivation can be invigorating, but as days turn into weeks, maintaining that momentum often becomes the real challenge. This is where technology can be your steadfast ally, bridging the gap between initial enthusiasm and long-term commitment. In today's fast-paced world, where schedules are packed to the brim, fitness apps offer a convenient and engaging solution to keep you accountable and motivated. These digital tools provide reminders, track progress, and even sprinkle in a bit of fun to keep you on track.

Fitness apps have become invaluable for those of us seeking to stay committed to our health goals amidst life's chaos.

They act as a personal coach tucked right in your pocket, guiding you with reminders and tracking your every step or calorie. Imagine having a virtual cheerleader that not only nudges you to get moving but also celebrates your accomplishments, big or small. Many apps seamlessly integrate with wearable devices, enhancing their effectiveness by providing real-time feedback on your activity levels. This integration allows you to set personalized goals and receive instant notifications, making it easier to stay informed and motivated. Whether you're running a marathon or simply aiming to increase your daily step count, these apps are designed to help you stay the course.

The concept of gamification in fitness apps takes motivation to another level. By introducing elements like reward systems and achievement badges, these apps make fitness feel less like a chore and more like a game. Imagine completing a workout and earning a badge that signifies your progress, or participating in virtual challenges that push you to achieve new milestones. These gamified elements tap into our innate desire to achieve and excel, transforming workouts into engaging and rewarding activities. Virtual competitions add an extra layer of excitement, allowing you to challenge friends or join global events, creating a sense of accountability and friendly rivalry that keeps you coming back for more.

When selecting the right fitness app, it's important to consider your personal goals and preferences. Start by evaluating the features each app offers—look for those that align with your fitness objectives and lifestyle. User reviews can provide valuable insights into the app's usability and effectiveness, helping you make an informed decision. It's also wise to try free versions of apps before committing to a paid subscription. This allows you to explore the interface, test the features, and determine whether the app truly meets your needs. Remember, the best app is one that seamlessly integrates into your daily routine, offering support and motivation without adding unnecessary complexity.

Interactive Journal: Fitness App Evaluation Checklist

- *Identify Your Goals: Determine your primary fitness objectives, such as weight loss, muscle gain, or increased endurance.*

- *Research Features: Look for apps with features that support your goals, such as workout plans, progress tracking, or social elements.*

- *Read User Reviews: Gain insights from other users regarding the app's effectiveness and usability.*

- *Test Free Versions: Try free versions or trial periods to evaluate the app's interface and features.*

- *Consider Integration: Ensure the app can sync with your wearable devices for enhanced tracking and engagement.*

- *Assess Community Aspects: Decide if social connectivity and community challenges are important to you in maintaining motivation.*

Digital Tools for Tracking Nutrition

Imagine standing in front of your pantry, trying to decide what to have for dinner. You want something nutritious, but after a long day, the last thing you want is to spend more time than necessary thinking about food. This is where digital tools for nutrition tracking come into play, simplifying the process of monitoring your dietary habits. With just a few taps on your smartphone, you can log your meals, scan barcodes for instant nutritional information, and even track your macro and micronutrient intake. These tools take the guesswork out of eating, allowing you to focus on enjoying your meals instead of worrying about them. Whether you're aiming to lose weight, maintain your current health, or reach new nutritional goals, these apps can provide the structure you need to stay on track.

Among the myriad of apps available, some stand out for their specific offerings. Lose It! is perfect for weight management, providing a straightforward platform to set goals and monitor your progress. It's user-friendly, with a database that helps you log foods quickly. If you're someone who needs detailed nutrient analysis, Cronometer is an excellent choice. It breaks down both macro and micronutrients, offering insights into your diet's nutritional profile and highlighting any deficiencies. For those who like to plan ahead, Yazio can be a game-changer. It not only helps you track what you eat but also assists in meal planning, catering to specific diets or preferences. By utilizing these apps, you gain access to a wealth of information that can help you make informed dietary choices tailored to your lifestyle and health needs.

Integrating nutrition data with your fitness goals can give you a comprehensive view of your health, allowing you to see how what you eat affects your physical performance. Many nutrition apps sync with fitness trackers, providing an all-encompassing picture of your daily activity and nutrition. By analyzing this data, you can adjust your dietary plans to better support your workouts, ensuring you're fueling your body appropriately. This integration fosters a deeper understanding of how your lifestyle choices interconnect, helping you make adjustments that lead to more balanced, effective health practices. When you see how your nutrition impacts your energy levels and workout recovery, you can tailor your meals to optimize performance and well-being.

Maintaining consistency in tracking can be a challenge, but with a few strategies, it becomes a sustainable habit. Setting daily reminders on your phone can prompt you to log meals and snacks consistently, making it part of your routine. Pre-logging meals can also help, especially if you have a regular eating schedule. By planning your meals ahead of time, you reduce the temptation to stray from your nutritional goals and ensure that you're prepared with healthy options. This approach not only keeps you accountable but also simplifies decision-making, reducing the stress associated with meal planning. The key is to find a rhythm that works for you, one that fits seamlessly into your daily life without feeling like a chore.

Interactive Element: Nutrition Tracking Reflection Prompt

Take a moment to reflect on your current approach to nutrition. Do you find yourself guessing what's in your meals, or do you have a system in place? Write down what you think works well and areas you'd like to improve. Then, consider how a digital tool could support your goals. Would it help with meal planning, nutrient tracking, or accountability? Identifying your needs can guide you to the right app, enhancing your nutritional habits with ease and precision.

Reflection on My Nutrition Tracking Take a moment to reflect on your current approach to nutrition. Do you find yourself guessing what's in your meals, or do you have a system in place? How do you track your food, if at all? How accurate or helpful do you find your current method?

What's Working Well Write down what you think works well in your current nutrition tracking. Are there any habits or tools that help you make healthier food choices?

Areas to Improve Reflect on areas where you feel your tracking could improve. Do you miss meals or forget to log certain items? Are there any gaps that leave you unsure about your nutrient intake?

The Role of Digital Tools Consider how a digital tool could support your goals. Would it help with meal planning, nutrient tracking, or accountability? How might an app streamline your process and make tracking easier?

Choosing the Right App Identify any needs or features that you would like a nutrition app to have. Would you prefer one with barcode scanning, meal suggestions, or nutrient breakdowns?

Small Steps to Improve Tracking What small steps can you take today to improve your nutrition tracking? Could you try a new app or make a habit of tracking after each meal?

Final Thoughts How does tracking your nutrition make you feel? What do you hope to achieve with a more structured approach to tracking your meals?

Music Suggestions Pair this reflection with soothing or motivational music for focus:

- *For Focus and Calm*: *Weightless* by Marconi Union

- *For Motivation and Clarity*: *Good Life* by OneRepublic

- *For Relaxation*: *Sunset Lover* by Petit Biscuit

Online Communities for Support and Motivation

Picture this: you've just completed a grueling workout, and while you feel accomplished, a part of you wishes you could share the moment with someone who truly gets it. Enter online communities—digital spaces that connect like-minded individuals who share your passion for wellness. These communities are more than just forums; they're hubs of support and motivation. They offer a unique blend of camaraderie and accountability, making your wellness journey less solitary and more social. Whether you're swapping workout tips, sharing personal victories, or seeking advice on overcoming challenges, these platforms cultivate a sense of belonging and encouragement.

One of the most vibrant online wellness communities is Reddit's fitness groups. It's a treasure trove of workout tips, advice, and personal stories that resonate with people from all walks of life. Whether you're a seasoned athlete or a fitness newbie, you'll find a wealth of information and inspiration here. App forums are another excellent resource, offering diet support and a chance to connect with others on similar health journeys. These forums are filled with individuals who understand the ups and downs of maintaining a healthy lifestyle, providing a safe space to share experiences and gain insights. Facebook groups focused on specific health goals also play a significant role in fostering supportive environments. From weight loss challenges to plant-based eating, there's a group for every interest, making it easy to find your tribe and stay motivated.

The power of peer support in achieving wellness goals cannot be overstated. Engaging with a community of like-minded individuals enhances accountability and persistence. When you witness others celebrating their successes, it fuels your motivation to keep pushing forward. Collaborative goal-setting becomes a shared endeavor, turning personal milestones into collective achievements. It's not just about ticking off a goal on your list; it's about doing it with the support and encouragement of others who want to see you succeed. This sense of community fosters resilience and commitment, making it easier to stay on track even when the going gets tough.

Finding the right online community can be a game-changer, but it's essential to choose one that aligns with your personal needs and values. Start by assessing the group's dynamics and culture. Are the interactions positive and supportive? Is there a sense of camaraderie and mutual respect? These factors are crucial in ensuring that the community will be a source of encouragement rather than stress. Explore multiple platforms to find the best fit for your goals and personality. Some people thrive in large, bustling forums, while others prefer smaller, more intimate spaces. Take the time to explore different options, and don't be afraid to leave a group if it doesn't feel right. The beauty of online communities lies in their diversity, offering countless opportunities to connect with people who share your passions and aspirations.

Remember, the value of these communities extends beyond immediate support. They provide a platform for lifelong learning and growth, where you can continually expand your knowledge and refine your approach to wellness.

Engaging with others introduces you to new perspectives and ideas, enriching your understanding of health and fitness. Whether it's discovering a new workout routine, learning about a different dietary approach, or simply finding inspiration in someone else's story, these interactions are invaluable. As you navigate your wellness journey, online communities can serve as a constant source of motivation and encouragement, reminding you that you're never alone in your pursuit of health and happiness.

Virtual Workouts: Finding What Works for You

Picture yourself at home, the day winding down, and you realize you haven't had the chance to exercise yet. Instead of feeling guilty for missing a gym session, you remember that you have an entire fitness studio at your fingertips. Virtual workouts have revolutionized how we approach exercise, offering a flexibility that fits seamlessly into our busy lives. They provide the convenience of at-home exercise, eliminating the need for travel and allowing you to work out on your schedule. With just a few clicks, you can access a diverse range of workout styles, from high-intensity interval training to calming yoga sessions, all from the comfort of your living room.

Platforms like Peloton have taken the fitness world by storm, known for their dynamic cycling and cardio classes that make you feel like you're part of a live studio session. The energy of the instructors and the community vibe can turn a regular workout into an exhilarating experience. If variety is what you crave, Beachbody On Demand offers an array of programs, ranging from intense strength training to dance-inspired routines, ensuring there's something for every mood and fitness level. For those seeking a more mindful approach, YogaGlo provides a sanctuary for yoga and meditation, helping you center your mind and body amidst life's chaos. These platforms cater to various preferences, making it easy to find workouts that resonate with your personal interests and fitness goals.

Exploring different workout styles not only keeps things fresh but also helps you discover what truly motivates you. Maybe you've always been a runner, but trying a dance cardio class brings a new level of joy to your routine. Or perhaps strength training has been your go-to, but incorporating some yoga helps balance your body and mind. Experimenting with various formats can reveal new passions and keep your fitness routine from becoming monotonous. It also allows you to adapt your workouts to changing goals. Whether you're training for a specific event, recovering from an injury, or simply seeking variety, the world of virtual workouts offers endless possibilities to tailor your exercise regimen.

Creating an effective virtual workout routine requires a bit of planning but can lead to a balanced and fulfilling fitness practice. Start by combining different types of workouts—strength, cardio, and flexibility—to ensure a well-rounded approach. This mix not only benefits your overall fitness but also keeps your body challenged and engaged. Setting regular workout times is crucial, as it establishes a routine that becomes a natural part of your day. Whether it's a morning session to kickstart your energy or an evening class to unwind, consistency is key. It's about finding a rhythm that suits your lifestyle, making exercise a habit rather than a chore.

To make the most of your virtual workouts, consider the environment where you'll exercise. Create a space that inspires movement, free from distractions and clutter. A simple mat, some weights, or resistance bands can transform any area into a mini gym. The goal is to cultivate a setting where you feel motivated and at ease, enhancing your focus and enjoyment of each session. As you explore the world of virtual workouts, remember that the journey is deeply personal. It's about discovering what moves you, both physically and emotionally, and embracing the freedom and flexibility that technology provides.

Mindfulness Apps to Enhance Meditation

Imagine starting your day with a few moments of quiet reflection, a time to set intentions and center yourself before the hustle and bustle begins. But finding the discipline to meditate consistently can be a challenge, especially when life feels like a whirlwind. Enter mindfulness apps, designed to help you establish and maintain a meditation routine that fits seamlessly into your daily life. These apps offer guided sessions perfect for beginners, taking the guesswork out of meditation and providing a gentle introduction to the practice. With the tap of a finger, you can access a library of meditations tailored to various needs and preferences, allowing you to explore different techniques and find what resonates most with you. Timer functions also cater to those who prefer self-paced practice, offering flexibility and autonomy in your meditation journey.

Among the array of apps available, some have gained popularity for their diverse meditation resources. Headspace is renowned for its structured learning approach, guiding users through meditation basics with ease and clarity. It's a great starting point for those new to mindfulness, offering step-by-step courses that build confidence and understanding. Calm, on the other hand, focuses on providing relaxation and sleep support, making it ideal for winding down after a long day. Its serene soundscapes and bedtime stories create a peaceful environment conducive to relaxation and rest. Insight Timer stands out with its extensive collection of meditations, catering to a wide range of styles and lengths. Whether you have a few minutes or an hour, Insight Timer offers something to suit your schedule and mood. Each app brings its unique strengths, allowing you to tailor your meditation experience to your personal needs and lifestyle.

Beyond the basics, mindfulness apps include features that enrich and deepen your meditation practice. Ambient sounds and music can transform your space into a tranquil retreat, enhancing the meditative experience and helping you focus. Many apps also offer progress tracking and milestones, allowing you to see your growth and stay motivated. As you reach milestones, such as consecutive days of meditation, you gain a sense of accomplishment and encouragement to continue. This progress tracking is more than just a record; it's a visual reminder of your commitment to self-care and inner peace. These features help maintain interest and engagement, making meditation a rewarding and evolving practice.

Incorporating meditation apps into your daily routine doesn't have to be complicated. Consider starting with a morning or evening ritual, dedicating a few minutes to mindfulness before the day begins or as it winds down. This routine can set a positive tone for your day or help you release the stress of daily life. If you find yourself overwhelmed during work, using an app for quick meditation breaks can provide relief and clarity, allowing you to return to tasks with renewed focus and calm. Integrate these moments of mindfulness into your schedule, treating them as essential as any other appointment or commitment. The key is consistency, finding a rhythm that complements your lifestyle and priorities.

Mindfulness apps serve as a bridge between intention and practice, offering tools and guidance to support your meditation journey. They provide a structure that makes meditation accessible to all, regardless of experience level. By incorporating these apps into your routine, you open the door to a world of mindfulness that can transform how you navigate life's challenges and joys. Whether you're seeking relaxation, focus, or personal growth, mindfulness apps offer a wealth of resources to accompany you on your path to self-discovery and tranquility.

Balancing Screen Time with Mindful Living

In today's digital age, screens have become an integral part of our lives, from smartphones and tablets to computers and televisions. While technology brings countless conveniences, it also presents challenges, especially when it comes to mental health. Excessive screen time can lead to digital fatigue, a condition characterized by symptoms such as eye strain, headaches, and mental exhaustion. It's easy to fall into the cycle of endless scrolling or binge-watching, only to find yourself feeling more drained than relaxed. Recognizing these symptoms is crucial for maintaining a healthy balance between technology use and mindfulness. Establishing boundaries around screen time is an effective way to mitigate these effects, ensuring that technology enhances rather than detracts from our well-being.

To foster mindful technology use, consider setting designated screen-free times throughout your day. These can be moments when you focus on activities that don't involve a screen, such as enjoying a meal with family, taking a walk, or engaging in a hobby. Creating these tech-free zones allows your mind to rest and recharge, reducing the cognitive load that constant screen interaction imposes. Additionally, apps designed to monitor and limit screen usage can be incredibly helpful. They provide insights into your screen time habits, helping you identify patterns and make conscious choices about when and how you use digital devices. By being aware of your screen time, you can take proactive steps to create a more balanced and mindful lifestyle.

Digital detox practices offer a refreshing break from the constant barrage of notifications and updates. Taking regular breaks from screens can significantly enhance your overall well-being. You'll likely notice increased focus and productivity as your mind becomes less cluttered with digital distractions. When you're not constantly switching between apps or web pages, you can concentrate more effectively on the task at hand. Improved sleep quality is another benefit of reducing screen time, especially before bed. The blue light emitted by screens can interfere with your natural sleep-wake cycle, making it harder to fall asleep and stay asleep. By limiting screen exposure in the evening, you create a more conducive environment for restful sleep, leading to better mental and physical health.

Creating a balanced digital lifestyle requires intentionality and commitment. Start by prioritizing offline activities that bring you joy and fulfillment. Whether it's reading a book, gardening, or spending time with loved ones, these activities offer meaningful engagement without the need for screens. Incorporating mindfulness practices into your daily routine can also help you stay grounded and present. This might involve simple breathing exercises, meditation, or just taking a moment to appreciate your surroundings. These practices encourage you to connect with the world around you, fostering a sense of peace and contentment that technology often disrupts. By making space for these moments, you nurture your mental health and cultivate a more balanced approach to technology use.

As you navigate the digital landscape, remember that the goal isn't to eliminate technology from your life but to use it mindfully and purposefully. By finding harmony between screen time and mindful living, you create a sustainable lifestyle that supports your well-being. This balance empowers you to enjoy the benefits of technology without becoming overwhelmed by its demands. With a conscious approach, you can harness the power of digital tools to enhance your life while maintaining a strong connection to the present moment and the world around you.

Chapter 9

Conclusion

As you reach the end of this journey through "Holistic Guide To Fitness," I hope you've found a friend in these pages, guiding you toward a more balanced and fulfilling lifestyle. We've explored the interconnectedness of mindful nutrition, holistic exercise, and sustainable weight loss, and how these elements work together to create a healthier you. Throughout the book, we've delved into the mind-body connection, emphasizing the importance of integrating mindfulness into your daily routines. This isn't just about counting calories or reps; it's about nurturing your entire self—mind, body, and spirit.

Let's take a moment to revisit the key insights we've uncovered. The benefits of connecting with your body and mind can't be overstated. Mindful eating transforms meals into moments of awareness and pleasure, helping you to savor each bite and understand your body's needs. Creating personalized fitness plans has empowered you to tailor your routines to fit your life, making exercise an enjoyable part of your day rather than a chore. We've tackled stress, revealing ways to manage it effectively through mindfulness and reflection.

The holistic approach we've advocated goes beyond traditional health advice. It's about adopting wellness practices that encourage self-reflection and growth. Through journaling, you've been invited to engage actively with the material, fostering self-awareness and personal development. This practice isn't just a task; it's a journey into understanding yourself better, uncovering what truly drives and fulfills you.

Now, it's time to take these strategies and techniques and weave them into the fabric of your everyday life. Consistency is key. Develop a routine that includes the exercises, meal plans, and mindfulness practices we've discussed. It might be setting aside time for a morning workout, preparing meals mindfully, or practicing deep breathing before bed. Whatever it is, make it yours.

You've been equipped with the tools to transform your life, and I encourage you to embrace this journey with confidence. Imagine the potential that lies ahead—a healthier, more vibrant you. Remember, transformation doesn't happen overnight. It's a gradual process, one that requires patience and persistence. But with each step, you move closer to the life you envision.

As you move forward, I invite you to join online communities and connect with others who share your goals. Share your experiences, learn from others, and find motivation in the stories of those who have walked this path before you. Use technology and apps to track your progress and maintain accountability. These tools can be your allies, helping you stay focused and inspired.

For ongoing support, keep an eye out for additional resources I may offer, be it through a website, app, or social media. These platforms can provide further guidance and updates, ensuring you're never alone in your wellness journey.

Thank you for trusting us and this book to guide you. Your commitment to your health and well-being is inspiring, and I'm confident that you have what it takes to achieve holistic wellness. Embrace this journey with an open heart and mind, knowing that every small step counts.

As you continue on this path, remember this: "The journey of a thousand miles begins with a single step." Live mindfully, cherish each day, and celebrate every victory, no matter how small. Here's to a healthier, happier you.

Extended Edition: Travel-Friendly Workouts

No gym? No problem. These zero-equipment circuits fit in any hotel room, park or small indoor space, keep your momentum on the road. Each circuit takes 8–15 minutes—just you, your bodyweight and common surfaces.

How to use

- Pick one circuit per session either morning, midday or evening

- Aim for 2–3 sessions on travel days; swap circuits to stay engaged

- Move at your own pace—rest 30 seconds between exercises or rounds

1 – Bodyweight Blast (10 minutes)

1. **Air Squats × 15**

   Stand with feet hip-width apart, toes pointing slightly outward. Hinge at the hips and bend your knees, lowering your hips back as if sitting into an invisible chair. Keep your chest lifted and weight in your heels. Drive through your heels to return to standing, squeezing glutes at the top.

2. **Incline Push-ups × 12**

   Place hands shoulder-width on a sturdy surface (bed or desk). Walk your feet back until your body forms a straight line from head to heels. Bend elbows to lower your chest toward the edge, keeping elbows at about 45°. Press through palms to straighten arms, bracing core throughout.

3. **Walking Lunges × 10 steps each leg**

   Step your right foot forward into a deep lunge, dropping your back knee toward the floor. Keep your front knee tracking over your ankle and torso upright. Push through the front heel to stand, then immediately step the left foot forward for the next lunge.

4. **Tricep Dips × 12**

   Sit on the edge of a chair, hands gripping the edge beside your hips. Slide your butt off the chair, legs extended in front. Lower your body by bending elbows until they reach about 90°, keeping shoulders down. Press through palms to straighten arms, engaging triceps.

5. **Mountain Climbers × 30 seconds**
Start in a high plank with hands beneath shoulders. Drive your right knee toward your chest, then quickly switch legs in a running motion. Keep hips steady and core tight—avoid sagging or piking.

Repeat 2 rounds

2 – Park Circuit (12 minutes)

1. **Bench Step-ups × 12 each leg**
Stand facing a bench or low wall. Place your right foot on the bench, press through your heel, and lift your body until your right leg is straight. Lower back slowly and switch legs.

2. **Push-ups on Bench × 10**
Hands on bench, feet on ground, body in straight line. Bend elbows to lower chest toward bench, keeping core braced. Press through palms to return.

1. **Bulgarian Split Squats × 10 each leg**
   Stand a couple of feet in front of the bench, place your rear foot on the bench's edge. Lower your front thigh until it's parallel to the ground, keeping front knee over ankle. Press through front heel to rise.

2. **Bench Plank × 30 seconds**
   Forearms on bench, feet on ground, body in a straight line. Squeeze glutes, draw belly button to spine, and hold without letting hips sag.

3. **Bench Jump-overs × 20 total**
   Stand to one side of bench. Bend knees, jump sideways over bench, landing softly on the balls of your feet with knees slightly bent. Repeat back.

Repeat 2 rounds

3 – Core & Balance Flow (8 minutes)

1. **Plank Shoulder Taps × 20 (10 per shoulder)**
   In high plank, feet wider than hip-width. Keeping hips stable, lift one hand to tap the opposite shoulder. Alternate sides, minimizing torso rotation.

2. **Single-Leg Deadlifts × 10 each leg**
   Stand tall, shift weight onto right foot. Hinge at hips, extend left leg straight back and reach hands toward

the floor. Keep back flat and shoulders square. Return to start and switch sides.

3. **Side Plank (Right) × 30 seconds**

   Lie on right side, forearm under shoulder, legs stacked. Lift hips until body forms a straight line. Hold, then switch sides.

4. **Side Plank (Left) × 30 seconds**

   Same form on your left side.

5. **Bird-Dog × 12 each side**

   On hands and knees, extend right arm forward and left leg back simultaneously. Keep hips level. Return and repeat with opposite limbs.

Perform as a straight set

4 – Stairs & Step Burn (15 minutes)

1. **Stair Run × 5 rounds**

   Sprint up a flight of stairs, using arms to drive. Walk back down for recovery.

2. **Calf Raises × 20**

   Stand on bottom stair edge, heels hanging off. Rise onto toes, pause, then lower until heels dip below step level.

3. **Incline Push-ups on Step × 12**

   Hands on bottom step, feet on ground. Keep body straight, lower chest to step, then press up.

4. **Decline Plank × 30 seconds**

   Feet on bottom step, hands on floor. Keep body rigid and core braced.

5. **Step Jump-ups × 10**

   Stand facing step. Bend knees, swing arms, and jump both feet onto step. Step down one foot at a time.

Repeat 2 rounds

5 – Express Upper-Body Pump (8 minutes)

1. **Push-ups × 12**

   Hands shoulder-width, body in straight line. Lower chest until elbows reach 90°, then press up.

2. **Chair Dips × 12**

   Hands on chair behind you, fingers facing forward. Lower hips until elbows bend 90°, then press up.

3. **Pike Push-ups × 10**

   From a "V" shape (hips high), bend elbows to lower head toward floor. Press back up, focusing on shoulder engagement.

4. **Reverse Plank × 30 seconds**

   Sit with legs extended, hands behind hips. Lift hips until body forms a straight line from head to heels.

5. **Arm Circles × 30 seconds each direction**

   Stand tall, arms out to sides. Make small circles forward for 30 seconds, then backward for 30 seconds.

Perform as a straight set

Sample Travel Day Plan

Morning – Wake-Up Charge
 – Bodyweight Blast (10 minutes)

Midday – Desk Detox
 – Core & Balance Flow (8 minutes)

Evening – Pre-Sleep Reset
 – Express Upper-Body Pump (8 minutes) + gentle full-body stretch (5 minutes)

Bonus Chapter: Fitness Myths Debunked

Separating Fact from Fiction

The world of fitness is full of information — some of it incredibly helpful, and some of it downright misleading. In this bonus chapter, we'll tackle some of the most common fitness myths and uncover the truths behind them to help you approach your fitness journey with confidence and clarity.

Introduction to the Bonus Chapter

Congratulations on reaching the conclusion of this book! As a special addition, this bonus chapter is designed to clear up common misconceptions that can hold you back or cause unnecessary confusion on your path to wellness. Let's get started on separating fact from fiction in the world of fitness.

Myth 1: Cardio is the Best Way to Lose Weight

The Truth: While cardio exercises like running and cycling are excellent for burning calories, they're not the only path to weight loss. Resistance training is equally important because it helps build muscle, which boosts your metabolism and leads to more calories burned even at rest. The best approach is a combination of both cardio and strength training for sustainable results.

Myth 2: Lifting Weights Makes Women Bulky

The Truth: This myth persists despite overwhelming evidence to the contrary. Women typically don't produce enough testosterone to gain massive muscle mass like men. Lifting weights can help women achieve a toned and sculpted physique, improve bone density, and enhance overall strength.

Myth 3: No Pain, No Gain

The Truth: While pushing yourself during workouts is important, pain is not a requirement for progress. Discomfort can signal effort, but sharp or persistent pain is your body's way of warning you about potential injury. Listen to your body and prioritize proper form and recovery to prevent setbacks.

Myth 4: You Can Target Fat Loss in Specific Areas

The Truth: Spot reduction, or targeting fat loss in specific areas through exercises, is a myth. When you lose fat, it happens across your entire body, not just the areas you work on. Consistent exercise, paired with a balanced diet, is the key to overall fat loss.

Myth 5: More Workouts Mean Faster Results

The Truth: Overtraining can actually hinder your progress and increase your risk of injury. Rest and recovery are essential components of any fitness routine. Muscles need time to repair and grow stronger, so incorporate rest days and prioritize sleep.

Myth 6: Stretching Before a Workout Prevents Injuries

The Truth: While stretching is important, static stretching (holding a stretch for a prolonged time) before a workout might not be the best choice. Dynamic warm-ups, which involve active movements that mimic your workout, are more effective in preparing your body and reducing the risk of injury.

Myth 7: You Need to Work Out Every Day to See Results

The Truth: Consistency is crucial, but quality matters more than quantity. A well-structured fitness routine with 3-5 days of focused exercise, complemented by active recovery and rest, can yield excellent results. Overworking yourself can lead to burnout and diminishing returns.

Myth 8: Crunches are the Best Way to Get Abs

The Truth: Crunches alone won't give you a six-pack. A strong core requires a mix of exercises that target different abdominal muscles, along with a healthy diet to reduce body fat. Planks, leg raises, and rotational movements are excellent additions to your core routine.

Myth 9: Eating More Protein Will Automatically Build Muscle

The Truth: Protein is vital for muscle repair and growth, but simply eating more protein without engaging in strength training won't lead to muscle gain. Pair your protein intake with resistance exercises to achieve optimal results.

Myth 10: Sweating More Means a Better Workout

The Truth: Sweating is your body's way of cooling down, not a measure of workout intensity or calorie burn. Factors like temperature, humidity, and individual differences influence how much you sweat. Focus on effort and proper technique rather than how much you sweat.

Myth 11: Fitness Requires Expensive Gym Memberships or Equipment

The Truth: You don't need a gym membership or fancy equipment to stay fit. Bodyweight exercises, outdoor activities, and affordable equipment like resistance bands can provide an effective workout. Fitness is about creativity and consistency, not cost.

Myth 12: Morning Workouts Are Better Than Evening Workouts

The Truth: The best time to work out is whenever you feel most energetic and can maintain consistency. Both morning and evening workouts have their advantages, so choose a time that aligns with your schedule and preferences.

Myth 13: Older Adults Should Avoid Strength Training

The Truth: Strength training is beneficial for people of all ages, including older adults. It helps maintain muscle mass, improve bone density, and enhance overall functionality, reducing the risk of falls and injuries.

Myth 14: If You're Not Sore, You Didn't Work Hard Enough

The Truth: Muscle soreness is not an accurate indicator of workout effectiveness. While some soreness is normal when trying new exercises, consistent training improves your recovery. Focus on progress in strength, endurance, and mobility instead.

Myth 15: Supplements Are Necessary for Fitness Success

The Truth: While some supplements can be helpful, they're not essential for achieving fitness goals. A balanced diet rich in whole foods can provide most of the nutrients you need. Consult a healthcare professional before adding supplements to your routine.

Final Thoughts

By dispelling these myths, you can approach fitness with a clearer understanding of what works and what doesn't. Remember, there's no one-size-fits-all approach to fitness. Listen to your body, embrace a balanced routine, and focus on long-term health rather than quick fixes.

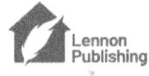

Thank You for Reading

We're so grateful you picked up *Holistic Living for Wellness*. We hope it brought you inspiration and practical tools for your wellness journey.

Enjoyed the book?

We'd love to hear your thoughts. Your review helps others discover the book and supports our growing wellness community.

Scan the QR code inside to leave a quick review, give us a like, or share your thoughts.

Every word you share means the world to us.

Thank you again for being part of this journey.

References

- Anderida Practice. (n.d.). *The holistic benefits of exercise for health and wellbeing*. Retrieved from https://www.theanderidapractice.com/news-all-posts/the-holistic-benefits-of-exercise-for-health-and-wellbeing

- Boss As A Service. (n.d.). *Using a workout accountability app to stick to your fitness plan*. Retrieved from https://bossasaservice.com/blog/workout-accountability-app/

- Business Insider. (n.d.). *Best mood trackers for mental health management*. Retrieved from https://www.businessinsider.com/guides/health/mental-health/mood-tracker

- Clear, J. (n.d.). *How to build new habits by taking advantage of old ones*. Retrieved from https://jamesclear.com/habit-stacking

- Clear, J. (n.d.). *How to master the art of continuous im-

provement. Retrieved from https://jamesclear.com/continuous-improvement

- Clear, J. (n.d.). *How to stick with good habits even when your willpower is low*. Retrieved from https://jamesclear.com/choice-architecture

- DFDRussell. (n.d.). *Digital detox: Managing screen time for better mental health*. Retrieved from https://www.dfdrussell.org/digital-detox-managing-screen-time-for-better-mental-health/

- EVŌLVE Strong. (n.d.). *Personalized fitness plans for better health*. Retrieved from https://evolvstrong.com/the-science-behind-custom-fitness-plans-why-personalization-leads-to-better-health-outcomes/

- Fitness CF Gyms. (n.d.). *Time-efficient workouts for busy lifestyles*. Retrieved from https://fitnesscfgyms.com/mountdorafl/blog/fitness-tips/time-efficient-workouts-for-busy-lifestyles/

- Graybiel, A. M. (2008). *The role of the basal ganglia in habit formation*. Nature Reviews Neuroscience, 7(6), 464-476. https://doi.org/10.1038/nrn1919

- Harvard T.H. Chan School of Public Health. (n.d.). *Healthy eating plate*. Retrieved from https://nutrition

source.hsph.harvard.edu/healthy-eating-plate/

- Healthline. (n.d.). *Mindful eating 101 — A beginner's guide*. Retrieved from https://www.healthline.com/nutrition/mindful-eating-guide

- Healthline. (n.d.). *The 8 best calorie counter apps*. Retrieved from https://www.healthline.com/nutrition/best-calorie-counters

- HumanGood. (n.d.). *7 low-impact exercises for older adults to stay active*. Retrieved from https://www.humangood.org/resources/senior-living-blog/low-impact-exercises-for-older-adults

- Johns Hopkins Medicine. (n.d.). *Hunger and fullness awareness*. Retrieved from https://www.hopkinsmedicine.org/health/wellness-and-prevention/hunger-and-fullness-awareness

- Mayo Clinic. (n.d.). *Mindfulness exercises*. Retrieved from https://www.mayoclinic.org/healthy-lifestyle/consumer-health/in-depth/mindfulness-exercises/art-20046356

- Mayo Clinic. (n.d.). *Positive thinking: Stop negative self-talk to reduce stress*. Retrieved from https://www.mayoclinic.org/healthy-lifestyle/stress

-management/in-depth/positive-thinking/art-20043950

- Mindful Leader. (n.d.). *7 breathing exercises for a balanced mind and body*. Retrieved from https://www.mindfulleader.org/blog/88637-harnessing-the-power-of-breath-7

- MindTools. (n.d.). *Visualization – Imagining and achieving your goals*. Retrieved from https://www.mindtools.com/a5ycdws/visualization

- National Center for Biotechnology Information. (2021). *Web workouts and consumer well-being: The role of digital fitness programs*. Retrieved from https://pmc.ncbi.nlm.nih.gov/articles/PMC8242656/

- National Center for Biotechnology Information. (2024). *Effects of mindfulness-based interventions on promoting mental health and well-being*. Retrieved from https://pmc.ncbi.nlm.nih.gov/articles/PMC9915077/#:~:text=In%20a%20Swiss%20study%20%5B33,helping%20them%20to%20perform%20better.

- Natural Resources Defense Council. (n.d.). *Industrial agricultural pollution 101*. Retrieved from https://www.nrdc.org/stories/industrial-agricul

tural-pollution-101

- Nutrition by Kristin. (n.d.). *100+ intuitive and mindful eating journal prompts from an intuitive eating dietitian.* Retrieved from https://nutritionbykristin.com/intuitive-and-mindful-eating-journal-prompts-from-an-intuitive-eating-dietitian/

- One Tree Planted. (n.d.). *9 tips for sustainable eating.* Retrieved from https://onetreeplanted.org/blogs/stories/9-tips-sustainable-eating

- Planet Forward. (n.d.). *Research shows plant-based diets better for your health.* Retrieved from https://planetforward.org/story/plant-based-diets-health/

- Positive Psychology. (n.d.). *5 benefits of journaling for mental health.* Retrieved from https://positivepsychology.com/benefits-of-journaling/#:~:text=Research%20suggests%20that%20expressive%20writing,lasting%20longer%20than%2030%20days.

- Tastewise. (n.d.). *Sustainable food sourcing: Data-driven strategies.* Retrieved from https://tastewise.io/blog/sustainable-food-sourcing#:~:text=Sustainable%20food%20sourcing%20is%20t he,local%20and%20small%2Dscale%20producers.

- United States Environmental Protection Agency. (n.d.). *Preventing wasted food at home*. Retrieved from https://www.epa.gov/recycle/preventing-wasted-food-home

- Verywell Mind. (n.d.). *Body scan meditation: Benefits and how to do it*. Retrieved from https://www.verywellmind.com/body-scan-meditation-why-and-how-3144782

- Wirecutter. (2025). *The 4 best meditation apps of 2025*. Retrieved from https://www.nytimes.com/wirecutter/reviews/best-meditation-apps/

www.ingramcontent.com/pod-product-compliance
Lightning Source LLC
Chambersburg PA
CBHW020541030426
42337CB00013B/939